THE RESET: STRONGER THAN BEFORE

Verses Kindler Publication

Verses Kindler Publication.

Website: www.verseskindlerpublication.com

Copyright & Terms of Use

From My Heart to Yours

The discernment shared in these pages are presented as a guide for self-discovery and mental fitness. It is essential to note that this book is not a medical manual, psychiatric guide, or clinical prescription for diet and fitness. The content reflects personal insights, lived experiences, and behavioural concepts related to long-term well-being.

Well-being is a deeply personal path influenced by genetics, history, and environment. As such, the concepts found here are illustrative and do not guarantee specific outcomes or health changes. This information should not be used to diagnose, treat, or prevent any medical condition.

Your safety is paramount. Please consult a physician or mental health practitioner to bridge these conceptions before altering your lifestyle. By reading on, you acknowledge that you are the ultimate steward of your own health and choices.

The Reset: Stronger Than Before
By: Kirti Jagasia
ISBN: 978-93-47494-46-8
1st Edition
Price: INR 299/$15

Disclaimer

The Reset: Stronger Than Before is authored by Kirti Jagasia. The entirety of this published work comprises the original content of the author, who has undertaken diligent efforts in its editing. The characters depicted herein may be fictitious or inspired by real events; however, they are not intended to cause offense or represent any prejudice against any caste or system. Any similarity to the names of actual individuals, locations, or institutions is purely coincidental and serves the narrative. The author bears sole responsibility for the originality of this work; the publisher assumes no liability thereof.

Contents

Dedication

To those who have tried to lose weight and found themselves starting over again and again, this book is for you.

It is for those who followed the plans, trusted the advice, and put in the effort, only to see the results fade. It is for those who quietly blamed themselves when things did not last, without recognizing how much discipline, patience, and strength they had already shown.

If you have ever stood in front of a mirror feeling disappointed, not because you didn't try, but because you didn't understand why it kept happening, these pages are meant for you. If you ever believed that you were the problem, this book hopes to help you see things differently.

Author's Note

My awareness of my body did not begin with the cold precision of a scale or the rigid rules of a diet plan. It began much earlier, in the quiet and formative years of adolescence; in those instinctive comparisons we make before we even have the words to describe them. Puberty arrived not only with physical change, but with an unspoken lesson: bodies are watched, judged, and constantly evaluated. Somewhere between growing taller and growing softer, I absorbed the belief that acceptance was not something we are born with, but something we must earn.

At first, this awareness was faint. A small noticing of how clothes fell on a friend, or how certain faces and bodies seemed to suit the camera better than others. But faint thoughts grow louder with time. Slowly, the message became clear: some bodies were seen as "right," while others were treated as projects in need of fixing. If your body didn't match the ideal, effort became your responsibility; your social cost.

That effort eventually led me into the world of dieting. I entered it with hope and sincerity. Diets promised order in a world filled with discomfort. They offered clarity, structure, and the comforting illusion of control. I followed the rules closely, trusted the experts, and believed that if I could just stay disciplined enough, I would finally find peace. For a short while, it worked. Early results bring a particular kind of pride; a brief sense of arrival, as though you've come home.

But the homecoming never lasted.

Each cycle followed the same painful rhythm: motivation, strict compliance, early success, and then the slow return to where I started. What hurt more than the weight coming back was the quiet loss of something deeper. With every failed attempt, a piece of confidence disappeared. Effort, once driven by hope, began to feel heavy and exhausting.

Repeated failure changes the way the mind works. Over time, the question shifts. It is no longer "Does this method work?" but "What is wrong with me?" You stop questioning the plan and start questioning your own character. The problem no longer feels like the map; it feels like the traveller. The exhaustion that follows is not just physical; it is emotional and spiritual. You are not only tired of trying. You are tired of believing.

In the process, I slowly lost touch with myself. I handed over my intuition to numbers and rules. I allowed spreadsheets to speak louder than my own body. Hunger, tiredness, and even joy stopped being signals to listen to and became problems to manage. I did not realise then that every attempt to control my body more tightly was damaging the very relationship I was trying to heal.

The real turning point did not arrive dramatically. It came quietly, like a slow dawn. I realised that chasing the "ideal" body was harming my mind far more than my weight ever had. The constant swing between pride and shame was leaving wounds that no fitness goal could fix. The true cost of this cycle added up over time, paid in lost clarity and broken self-trust.

When I looked at the fitness industry to reflect on this experience, I found little recognition. The industry speaks fluently about transformation, discipline, and grit, but struggles with empathy. It often treats struggle as weakness and relapse as failure. It celebrates results while ignoring the emotional damage left behind. It is an industry focused on outcomes, rarely pausing to consider the human experience along the way.

This book was not written to trap you in another set of rules or to fix a body that was never broken. It was written to quiet the constant mental noise around food, movement, and self-worth.

It exists because too many people are carrying the burden of a system that was designed to fail them, blaming themselves for paths that led nowhere. Understanding is not a consolation prize; it is the foundation on which real change is built.

What follows is not a roadmap. It is not a promise. It is an exploration of the invisible forces, beliefs, pressures, and patterns that shape our relationship with health. Before discipline can be built, trust must be restored.

This book does not begin with change.

It begins with understanding.

Introduction: Why This Book Exists

Have you ever noticed how your phone seems to know exactly when you're feeling "off"? You're scrolling, perhaps in a quiet moment of self-doubt, and there it is: a miracle supplement, a 30-day "shred," or a fitness guru explaining why your morning coffee is the reason you haven't reached your goals.

Advice is everywhere. It's in our group chats, on our bedside tables, and echoing in our heads every time we look in the mirror. *Eat this. Avoid that. Wake up at 5:00 a.m. Be disciplined. Trust the process.* And then comes the familiar, whispered prayer we offer ourselves after a long day: *It's okay. I'll start again on Monday.*

Monday is the great reset button. It's our way of forgiving the week that didn't go as planned. But as Mondays turn into months, a quiet exhaustion sets in. The body gets tired, yes, but it's the mind that truly burns out. For many of us, this struggle didn't begin with a diet. It began in the hallways of adolescence.

Think back to that age when you first noticed the world changing, and the world noticed you. Classmates changed. Curves appeared. Compliments followed for some, while silence followed for others. Almost instinctively, you began to keep score. You compared marks, complexion, height, and achievements. Slowly, the comparison leaked into every corner of your identity. Puberty is meant to be a phase of growth, but when hormones meet high expectations, it becomes an emotional gauntlet. When the body doesn't match the "ideal" being rewarded on screen or in class, the mind draws a devastating conclusion: *Something is wrong with me.* That belief hits early and hard.

From that moment on, weight loss stops being about health. It becomes a verdict. A test you feel you've failed before you even step into the arena. To compensate, we try harder. We overdo. We chase validation like its oxygen.

This is where the shortcuts start to look like lifelines. The shakes, the crash diets, the "instant" programs; they work, for a moment. The scale drops. The compliments flood in. For a few weeks, you feel untouchable.

And then, inevitably, the weight returns. Sometimes it brings friends.

But what returns with the weight is far more dangerous: the disappointment, the self-hatred, and the crushing realisation that you can no longer trust your own word.

Here is the part the multi-billion-dollar industry rarely speaks about: Most weight-loss attempts damage our mental health far more than the actual weight we carry. This cycle of "hope, success, and collapse" rewires our brains. It creates an addiction to instant results and a dangerous tolerance for denial. We become willing to ignore health risks just for the high of a temporary win. It is eerily similar to a volatile stock market, except in the markets, you only risk your money. Here, you are gambling with your life.

The industry grows while we shrink; not in size, but in spirit. Studies show that 80–95% of diets fail. Not because you lack willpower, but because the emotional cost of the "restart" is never addressed.

Most books focus on the plate or the gym. This book focuses on the space between your ears. Because when the mind is exhausted, even the "perfect" plan is just another burden you aren't ready to carry.

This book exists to bridge that gap.

- It is not a diet book.
- It is not a fitness routine.

- It offers no shortcuts, because you've already taken enough of them.

Instead, it offers clarity. We are going to explore how your beliefs were formed, why pressure builds until you snap, and how confusion, not a lack of effort, is what's truly keeping you stuck.

You don't need another Monday. You need a new lens. This isn't a book about losing weight.

It's a book about losing the confusion.

PART I: WHERE IT ALL BEGINS: MIND & CONDITIONING

When Weight Became a Verdict

There was a golden, unscripted era in life when the body did not require a defence attorney. In the hazy landscape of early childhood, the body existed as a kind of biological playground; a vessel to run with, tumble through the day in, and forget entirely the moment sleep arrived. We moved until our lungs burned simply because movement felt like electricity. We ate when hunger announced itself with a roar and stopped the second satisfaction settled in like a quiet hum. Back then, the body was a neutral, reliable partner. You didn't "watch" your body; you simply were your body. You didn't look in the mirror to check for flaws or judge yourself. You only looked to see if you had chocolate on your face or to show off a scrape from playing outside. But somewhere along the journey toward adulthood, that neutrality vanished. It wasn't a sudden, violent crash, but a gradual, humid shift; a moment in front of a mirror when the body stopped being a home and started becoming a performance.

I remember standing before a mirror, its wooden frame chipped and peeling, never designed to carry the heavy, suffocating weight of self-scrutiny. I was young, still growing, still very much a work in progress. By any medical definition, I was healthy. My body was doing exactly what bodies are programmed to do during that volatile phase of life. Yet, every change felt amplified, as if a magnifying glass had been placed over my insecurities. Because I was short, every slight shift in my silhouette felt like a seismic event. While my peers seemed to stretch upward into graceful lines, I felt like I was expanding outward in ways I hadn't given permission for.

The Verdict

My attention narrowed into a single, unforgivable point: the soft curve of my belly. It wasn't my hips or my thighs that bothered me yet; it was that small, stubborn arc of flesh that appeared when I sat down. I remember the tactile sensation of it; I would pinch the skin between my thumb and forefinger, watching it yield and spring back, silently demanding to know why I couldn't just remain "flat" or "normal." I'd suck my breath in until my ribs ached, trying to see if I could make that version of myself permanent. Without realising it, that was the moment the trial began. Weight stepped in as the verdict, shaping not only how I looked in a pair of jeans, but the very core of who I believed I was allowed to be.

Guest in My Own Skin

As that obsession took hold, it began to rewrite my inner narrative with a cruel, steady hand. Adolescence arrives like a trespasser in the night, stealing our bodily innocence and replacing it with a sharp, unrelenting lens of comparison. Suddenly, your value feels conditional. You start to believe that acceptance is a prize awarded only to those who mirror an unspoken, airbrushed ideal. For those of us who aren't necessarily "overweight" by a scale's standards, but who feel persistently, naggingly "imperfect," the anxiety is particularly insidious. There is no obvious "problem" to solve, no medical intervention required; only a lingering, poisonous sense of not being quite right. You begin to feel like a stranger in your own body, constantly wondering if you are 'good enough' to belong among the attractive people.

This external pressure collides head-on with an internal revolution that no one prepares you for. Puberty is not a subtle guest; it is a riot. Hormones surge, redistributing fat to places that feel alien, accelerating growth in bursts that leave you clumsy and disconnected. Biology understands this as a necessary preparation for adulthood, but from the inside, it feels like a profound betrayal. Just as the world starts demanding we be sharper and more controlled, our bodies do the opposite—they begin to soften and round. Because I had a small frame, these natural developments felt like an invasion. My reflection no longer matched the image I believed I needed to present to be taken seriously.

I didn’t have the language back then to understand that my brain was also undergoing a massive restructuring. I didn't know that my emotional volume had been turned up to the max, or that social cues, a half-smile from a classmate or a whispered joke in the hallway, registered as deafening shouts of rejection. Without a biological map to guide me, I interpreted the miracle of growth as a personal failure of character. I looked at the softening of my jawline or the widening of my waist and saw a lack of "grit." I saw apathy and slovenliness where there was actually just life. Slowly, a dangerous myth took root: the idea that body size is a direct reflection of a person’s soul. I began to believe that thinness was shorthand for success, intelligence, and morality, while any deviation was a sign of a weak will. This belief is a pollutant in the air we breathe; reinforced through every movie where the "hero" is lean and the "sidekick" is the punchline.

We absorb these stories long before we have the tools to question them. We are taught to ignore the vast, invisible systems of genetics, metabolism, and bone structure, and instead, assign all the blame to willpower. We are trained to view "small" as "good" and "restriction" as a virtue. We turn our daily lives into a constant act of self-surveillance, checking the "fit" of our clothes every hour as if our worth might have expired since breakfast.

Living in the Waiting Room

Once comparison enters the room, discomfort usually follows and settles in for the long haul. In school hallways, social circles, and even cafeteria lines, eating becomes a public performance rather than a private necessity. I remember watching friends eat pizza or fries with an enviable, breezy freedom, while I sat back, mentally calculating the "cost" of every bite. I would negotiate with myself: If I eat this now, I won't eat dinner later. Pleasure became a debt that had to be paid back with interest. Even a moment of genuine enjoyment felt suspicious, as if the mere act of wanting food was a crime that would eventually be punished by the mirror.

This shame isn't always born from cruelty; often, it's the "afterthought" feelings that hurt the most. It's the way you feel after a group photo is taken, when everyone crowds around the phone to see how they look, and you feel a physical jolt of nausea at the sight of your own arm or the way your chin looks at that specific angle. You smile through the discomfort, but inside, you are already planning how to hide better next time. These moments teach the body to shrink, not just physically, but energetically. You stop raising your hand; you stop wearing bright colours; you stop being "loud." You become a master of the "side-angle" and the "oversized hoodie," trying to occupy as little space as possible so as not to offend the eyes of others.

Family spaces, which should be our ultimate sanctuary, are often the places where these scripts are most deeply etched. Even the most well-meaning comments, "Are you sure you want seconds?" or "That shirt is a bit tight, isn't it?"; land like lead in the stomach of a sensitive teenager. These gestures, often born out of a parent's own internalised fear or their desire to "protect" us from the world's judgment, actually do the opposite. They communicate a devastating message: your body is a problem to be managed, not a home to be trusted. You learn that love and approval are things you have to maintain through constant vigilance. You start to use humour as armour, making the "fat joke" about yourself before anyone else can, hoping that if you deliver the verdict first, the sentence won't be as heavy.

By the height of adolescence, weight stops being a physical characteristic and becomes a permission slip. We begin to live life in the "waiting room." We tell ourselves we will go to the beach, apply for that job, or finally talk to our crush once we lose five pounds. We put our joy on layaway, waiting for a version of ourselves that doesn't exist to show up and give us the "okay" to start living. We treat our happiness like a luxury we haven't earned yet, convinced that we must pay a "toll" of pounds or inches before we deserve to participate in our own lives. We are essentially holding our breath, stalling our potential and pausing our memories in exchange for a "perfect" tomorrow that never arrives. We stay on the sidelines of our own existence, saving the best parts of ourselves for a future body that is always just out of reach. Because of this, we miss out on the cold sting of the ocean and the heat of a summer bonfire, too busy wondering if our thighs look "huge" in our shorts. We are physically present, but mentally, we are miles away, locked in a boardroom meeting with our insecurities. But the truth, the quiet, unsettling, and ultimately beautiful truth, is that the trial was rigged from the start. The verdict of "unforgivable" that we gave ourselves was based on a fundamental misunderstanding of what a body is for. The body was never meant to be a statue to be admired; it was meant to be a vehicle for experience. Our willpower was blamed for biological processes that were entirely out of our conscious control. Our character was judged against standards designed by industries that profit from our dissatisfaction. Healing does not begin with "fixing" the body or finally reaching that goal weight that we think will solve our problems. It doesn't begin with a new diet or a more rigorous exercise plan. It begins with the radical realisation that the accusation itself was flawed. We spend years defending ourselves against the charge of being "too much" or "not enough," never stopping to ask who wrote the law we are supposedly breaking. We realise that we are being prosecuted for the "crime" of having a body that changes, ages, and breathes; a crime that is actually just the evidence of being alive. The case against us was built on hollow evidence and impossible standards, meant to keep us distracted and ashamed. It begins when we look at that chipped mirror and realise that the person staring back isn't a criminal on trial, but a human being who has been trying to survive in a world that taught them to hate their own home. The first step toward freedom is refusing to show up for the court date anymore.

The First Defence

If you are reading this and feeling that familiar ache in your chest, the "Oh, they're talking about me" feeling, I want you to know something. There was a time when your body didn't need defending. This chapter isn't here to give you a meal plan or a workout routine. We have enough of those. It is here to help you recognise that the trial you've been living in was rigged from the start. You've been blaming your willpower for a biological process. You've been blaming your character for a cultural myth. Before anything can change, the verdict has to be recognised for what it is: a misunderstanding. As Naomi Wolf nailed it in The Beauty Myth (1990): "Pain is perfect cover for social control."

Pause & Notice (15 seconds)

I want you to close your eyes. Don't analyse your day. Don't judge what you ate for lunch. Just take a breath and ask yourself quietly: "When did my body stop feeling neutral?" Was it a comment? A mirror? A locker room? A family dinner? Hold that moment gently. Notice the echo it leaves in your chest. You don't need to fix it yet. You don't even need to know what to do with it. Just notice. Because this is where the trial began... and this is where healing whispers its very first defence.

The Psychology of Daily Failure

It's 7:00 AM on a Saturday. You've had a "perfect" week. You've swapped your morning croissant for overnight oats that look (and occasionally taste) like wet cement. You've walked 10,000 steps every day, tracking them with the fervour of a private investigator. You even turned down the office pizza on Thursday, a feat of heroism that surely deserves a small parade.

Confident and humming a little tune, you step onto the scale. You wait for the digital numbers to flash. You're expecting a landslide; a transformation so profound the scale might actually thank you.

The numbers stop blinking. You've gained 300 grams.

In that moment, something breaks. It isn't just your heart; it's your psychological contract with "The Journey." You look at the scale, then at your reflection, and then at the trash can where those oats belong. This is the Psychology of Daily Failure, a mental landscape where logic goes to die and the "What the Hell" effect takes over. Within twenty minutes, you're knee-deep in a bag of salt-and-vinegar chips because, hey, if the "good" life isn't working, the "bad" life might as well be delicious.

The Silent Scream

We live in a world of "On-Demand" everything. If your Netflix takes more than three seconds to buffer, you're ready to call your internet provider and demand a refund. We are conditioned for a 1:1 ratio of Input to Output.

However, your biology is not a vending machine. You cannot simply insert one salad and receive one visible ab.

The Sacrifice of the "Half-Informed"

You are at an age where the world is full of "interesting" things to eat; cravings and attractions are at their peak, yet you deny yourself every single one. You sacrifice the joy of the present for the promise of a different future. However, because you are operating with half-information and a lack of awareness regarding what is actually "good" or "bad" intake, you default to extremes. In the blind fear of gaining weight, you avoid everything, even the nutrients your body desperately needs to function. You put in 100% effort, but because the strategy is built on deprivation rather than data, the scale refuses to move the next morning. This isn't just a physical plateau; it is the breeding ground for frustration that inevitably turns into overeating and self-destruction.

When you start a health transformation, you are essentially trying to turn around a massive oil tanker with a small wooden paddle. You are paddling like crazy. You are sweating. You are exhausted. But if you look at the horizon, the ship still seems to be heading toward "Heartburn Island."

This is the most dangerous phase of any change: The Gap. It's the space between your effort and your evidence. Most people quit in The Gap because their brain tells them a very convincing lie: *"If you can't see it, it isn't happening."* But beneath the surface, your cellular machinery is frantic. Your mitochondria are waking up, your insulin sensitivity is shifting, and your liver is finally getting a break from processing high-fructose corn syrup. You're winning the war; you just haven't captured the capital city yet.

The Fatigue Illusion

We often mistake failure for a lack of physical stamina, but the true culprit is emotional fatigue. It's the exhaustion of saying "no" to your cravings all day while saying "yes" to a relentless boss. This mental drain lowers your physical pain threshold; the world literally feels heavier because your brain has lost its "buffer" for discomfort. When you are emotionally depleted, you don't just feel tired; you feel defeated. You begin to identify with the failure rather than the struggle. You aren't just "someone trying to be healthy"; you become "someone who always fails," and that identity is a heavier weight than any physical poundage.

Let's talk about why you're *actually* tired.

There is a biological limit to how much "no" your brain can say in a single day. Psychologists call this Ego Depletion. Imagine your willpower is like a smartphone battery.

- 7:00 AM: 100%. You say "no" to the snooze button. (Battery: 95%)
- 9:00 AM: You say "no" to the cream in your coffee. (Battery: 85%)
- 1:00 PM: You say "no" to the pasta and "yes" to the wilted arugula. (Battery: 60%)
- 4:00 PM: Your boss sends a passive-aggressive email. (Battery: 15%)
- 6:00 PM: You walk past a bakery. (Battery: 2%)

By understanding that your legs and hands are capable, you can shift from feeling physically defeated to appreciating your body's efforts. This awareness builds confidence and encourages continued effort.

We often think failure is a lack of physical stamina. It's not. It's a lack of mental bandwidth. When we fail daily, it's usually because we try to fight too many battles with a low battery. We blame our bodies for being weak when we should be blaming our schedules for being relentless.

How Repeated Failure Rewires Your Confidence

Every time you tell yourself, "Starting Monday, I'm a new person," and then by Wednesday you're eating leftover cake over the sink, you are performing a tiny, accidental lobotomy on your own self-trust.

Confidence isn't a personality trait; it's a track record.

If a friend constantly promised to pick you up from the airport and never showed up, you'd eventually stop asking them. When you constantly break promises to yourself, your brain treats you like that flaky friend. It stops believing you.

This leads to the "Rewired for Defeat" state. You start a new plan, but a voice in the back of your head whispers, *"Don't get too excited, we both know how this ends."* You begin to identify with the failure rather than the struggle. You aren't "someone who is learning to be healthy"; you become "someone who always fails." This identity is the heaviest weight you'll ever have to lose.

Did You Know?

Mental fatigue actually lowers your physical pain threshold. In studies, participants who completed difficult mental puzzles before exercising reported feeling "the burn" much sooner than those who hadn't. When your mind is tired, the world literally feels heavier. Your 5kg dumbbells start feeling like 10kg because your brain has lost its "buffer" for discomfort.

Why the "Journey" Stops Being a Journey

The fitness industry loves the word "Journey." It sounds like a spiritual pilgrimage through the Himalayas. But let's be honest: for most of us, it feels like being stuck in a suburban traffic jam.

The "Journey" stops being fun when it becomes a metric-driven obsession. When the only thing that matters is the number on the scale, the number on your bicep, or the number on your sleep tracker, you aren't on a journey anymore; you're an accountant for your own body.

And let's be real: nobody likes accounting.

We lose the joy of movement because we're too busy calculating the caloric "repayment" for a slice of bread. We stop appreciating the fact that we can breathe deeply, walk fast, or carry groceries without gasping. The "Journey" becomes a treadmill; constant motion, high anxiety, and the scenery never changes. We become obsessed with the "After" photo, forgetting that we have to live in the "During" for the rest of our lives.

The Speed Paradox: Jet vs. Snail

Everything in your life revolves around immediate results. We are young, dynamic, and living in a world that moves at the speed of a jet. Your corporate career demands rapid growth and instant pivots. But while your professional life is flying, your weight loss journey is moving like a snail. It is incredibly difficult to find balance when you are expected to be a high-performer at work while feeling like a low-performer in your own skin. When the gap between your career velocity and your biological progress becomes too wide, the "journey" stops being a path to health; it becomes a failed mission. This misalignment is where the seeds of depression are sown.

I spent years thinking that "Discipline" was a hammer you used to beat yourself into submission. I thought if I didn't feel bad about my failures, I wouldn't change. I recently figured out that shame is the worst fuel for change. Shame is a high-octane fuel that burns out your engine in ten minutes. It makes you hide. It makes you avoid the scale. It makes you lie to your trainer.

The people who actually transform aren't the ones who are hardest on themselves; they are the ones who are the most curious. Instead of saying, *"I failed because I'm lazy,"* they say, *"That's interesting. I ate that whole pizza because I hadn't eaten lunch, and I was stressed. Maybe next time I'll have a snack at 3:00 PM."* When you swap Judgment for Curiosity, the "Daily Failure" stops being a tragedy and starts being data. And you can't argue with data.

The Instagram Hallucination

We cannot talk about the psychology of failure without mentioning the glowing rectangle in your pocket. Comparing your "Day 2" to someone else's "Year 10" is like comparing a sapling to an oak tree and being mad that the sapling doesn't provide shade. We see "influencers" who seem to live in a perpetual state of hydration and sunlight, never failing, never bloating, and apparently never eating anything that wasn't grown in a volcanic mineral spring. This creates a "False Baseline." We think their "extraordinary" is "normal," which makes our "normal" feel like "failure."

Comparison is the thief of joy, but it's also the architect of frustration. Your body is playing a different game than theirs. You have different stressors, different gut bacteria, and a different history. Failing to look like a filtered image isn't a failure; it's just reality.

The Power of the "Non-Scale Victory"

To survive the psychology of daily failure, we need a new currency. If the scale is a "Mean Boss" who refuses to give you a raise, you need to start looking for the "Under-the-table" benefits.

- Did you have the energy to stay awake during that 2:00 PM meeting? Win.
- Did you choose water once when you really wanted soda? Win.

- Did you put on a pair of jeans and realise you didn't have to do "The Jump and Wiggle" to get them over your hips? Massive Win.

When we broaden our definition of success, "Daily Failure" starts to evaporate. You realise that while the scale is stagnant, your life is actually expanding.

The Mirror Question:

Tomorrow morning, when you look in the mirror, try to ignore the "imperfections" for exactly sixty seconds. Instead, ask yourself: "What did this body do for me today?" Did it carry you to work? Did it allow you to hug someone? Did it digest your food without you having to think about it?

Awareness Note:

Failure is rarely a permanent state; it's usually just a temporary feeling caused by a mismatch between your expectations and your biology. Your body isn't fighting against you; it's just busy doing a million things you can't see.

The only real failure is stopping the clock. As long as the clock is ticking and you're still curious, you're still in the game.

Why Weight Loss Hurts the Mind First

If you've ever stood in front of a mirror, pulling at the waistband of pants that fit three weeks ago but are currently staging a protest, you know the feeling. It's not just being "bummed out." It's a specific, hollow ache in the centre of your chest. It's the feeling of a promise broken: not by a lying politician, a shady mechanic, or a flaky friend, but by the person you're supposed to trust most: yourself.

We are force-fed a narrative that weight loss is the ultimate "glow-up." The marketing machine promises that as the numbers on the scale go down, your charisma will skyrocket, your career will flourish, and your zest for life will reach heights previously reserved for people in yoghurt commercials. But for millions of us, the exact opposite happens. The process of chronic dieting doesn't just burn fat; it often incinerates our mental well-being, leaving behind a version of ourselves that is thinner, perhaps, but also quieter, sadder, and profoundly lonely.

Welcome to the psychological "underbelly" of the weight-loss industry. Grab a coffee (the full-fat kind, please: we need the brain fuel), because we're going to talk about why weight loss often hurts the mind long before it ever helps the body.

1. Dieting as Psychological Injury: The Hope-Collapse Cycle

In physics, there is a concept called "material fatigue." It describes what happens when you take a sturdy piece of metal and bend it back and forth, over and over. At first, it stays strong. Then, micro-cracks form. Eventually, it snaps: not because the last bend was particularly hard, but because the structural integrity has been compromised by repeated stress.

Your psyche works the same way. Every time you start a new diet, you experience a "Hope Spike." You buy the meal-prep containers, the neon sneakers, and those $40 tubs of "superfood" powder that tastes like chalk and regret, the kind that quietly sell in India for the price of a week's groceries. This isn't just a financial transaction; it's an emotional investment. You are betting your happiness on a new version of you. But when the plan eventually fails: usually because it was biologically unsustainable, not because you lack "willpower": the collapse isn't just a physical return to your old weight. It's a psychological injury.

Behavioural psychology calls this the erosion of self-trust. After the fourth or fifth cycle, your brain stops believing you when you say, "This time is different." You start associating the very idea of self-improvement with pain, deprivation, and inevitable rejection. You aren't just failing a diet; you're witnessing a slow-motion car crash of your self-identity. You move from being "someone who is trying" to "someone who is fundamentally broken."

2. Depression Without Sadness: The Big Numb

When we think of depression, we think of the Hollywood version: weeping in bed, sad music, and unwashed hair. But diet-related depression is often much stealthier. It is a state called anhedonia: the loss of the ability to feel pleasure.

Have you ever been three weeks into a restrictive regime and realised you just… don't care about anything? Your favourite hobby feels like a chore. Your partner's jokes aren't funny. You aren't "sad" in the traditional sense; you're just *grey*.

This is "Atypical Depression" sparked by mental fatigue. Your brain is under so much "cognitive load" from tracking macros, weighing protein, and resisting the bread basket that it shuts down non-essential emotional functions to save energy. You aren't living; you're managing a spreadsheet. Research into "Cognitive Load Theory" suggests that when we overtax our executive function with constant self-monitoring, our emotional regulation and capacity for joy are the first things to go. You become a "Human Doing" instead of a "Human Being."

3. Shame-Induced Isolation: The "I'll Go When I'm Ready" Trap

Weight regain doesn't just hurt your ego; it shrinks your world. It starts with the "No."

- *"Want to go to the beach?"* No, I don't have a suit that hides the ten pounds I put back on.
- *"Want to go to the high school reunion?"* No, I'll wait until I'm back to my 'goal size' so I don't have to explain why I look like this.
- *"Want to try that new dating app?"* Not yet. Maybe in three months, when I've "fixed" this.

This is Body-Based Shame, and it is a social poison. We treat our bodies like a ticket to entry for society. If we don't have the ticket, we don't go to the show. Research shows that social isolation is as damaging to health as smoking 15 cigarettes a day. Ironically, by trying to get "healthy" through shameful dieting, we often end up in a state of loneliness that is physically and mentally more dangerous than the weight itself. We stop being participants in our own lives and become spectators, waiting for a "better body" to permit us to show up.

Myth vs. Reality

The Myth: Weight loss builds permanent confidence.

The Reality: Confidence built on a number is conditional. If your self-worth is tied to a result you can't perfectly control (like the fluctuating weight of a biological organism), your confidence is a house of cards. True confidence is built on self-efficacy: the belief that you can take care of yourself and remain kind to yourself regardless of what the scale says.

4. The Dragon Scroll Illusion

In the movie *Kung Fu Panda*, the hero, Po, spends the entire story obsessed with the "Dragon Scroll": a legendary artefact said to grant "limitless power" to whoever reads it. The villain is willing to kill for it. Po is willing to die for it.

When Po finally opens the scroll, his heart sinks. The scroll is blank. It's just a piece of reflective gold paper.

This is the perfect metaphor for the "Goal Weight." We are told that reaching a specific size is the secret scroll that will unlock our "real" lives. We think, *"When I'm a size 10, I'll finally be the confident, happy version of me."* But when people hit that number, they often find the scroll is blank. They realise they are the same person, with the same anxieties, just in a smaller pair of jeans.

The "limitless power" wasn't in the secret hacks, the fasting windows, or the restrictive formulas; it was in the realisation that the reflection in the scroll was enough all along. The industry sells you the scroll, but they never tell you that the magic is supposed to be *you*, not the paper.

5. Why Confidence Collapses When Weight Returns

If you lose weight through self-hate, you're building your foundation on a swamp. When the weight inevitably returns, which it does for the vast majority of people because of biological "set-point" defences, the confidence doesn't just "dip"; it structurally erodes.

This leads us to Martin Seligman's theory of Learned Helplessness. In his research, subjects who were repeatedly exposed to adverse outcomes they couldn't control eventually stopped trying altogether: even when a solution was right in front of them.

After enough diet cycles, your brain decides that effort is useless. You don't just think "the diet failed"; you think "I am a failure." You stop saying "I'll try again" and start asking "What's the point?" This shift from *effort-based thinking* to *identity-based brokenness* is the most expensive cost of dieting. It's the loss of the "future self" you used to believe in.

6. The Cost Nobody Talks About: The Mental Tax

Dieting is a massive Emotional Labour tax. We only have a finite amount of mental energy each day. Think about the bandwidth it takes to:

1. Constantly monitor your hunger signals and then actively ignore them.
2. Calculate the "social cost" of every dinner invitation.
3. Manage the perceived "public failure" of your body changing.

This leads to a "smaller" life. You become more rigid, less spontaneous, and, honestly, more judgmental. When you are starving and strict with yourself, it is almost impossible not to look at others with a critical eye. You trade your joy, your creativity, and your spontaneity for a temporary, fleeting sense of control.

7. Reclaiming the Mind

We have been taught that the "mental" part of weight loss is just "discipline." That is a lie. The mental part of health is actually Self-Compassion and Resilience. If you are currently in the "grey" zone: feeling numb, isolated, or like you've lost your "spark" because of the constant battle with food, know that this is a physiological response to psychological trauma. Your brain is trying to protect you from the pain of another "Hope-Collapse" cycle by making you care less.

The way out isn't a better diet. It's rebuilding the self-trust that the industry broke. It's realising that your value is not a fluctuating variable based on gravity's pull on your body.

15-Second Emotional Self-Check

Before you turn the page, take a breath. Just one. Close your eyes for 15 seconds and ask yourself these three questions. Don't try to fix the answers; just notice them like you're watching clouds pass by.

1. The Voice: If I spoke to my best friend the way I speak to myself in the mirror, would I still have a best friend?
2. The Trust: On a scale of 1-10, how much do I actually trust my body to tell me what it needs right now?
3. The Space: If I stopped thinking about my weight tomorrow, what would I do with all that extra "brain space"? What hobbies or dreams have I been putting off?

If you feel a sense of grief or perhaps a heavy silence answering these, you aren't a failure. You are simply someone who has been fighting a war you weren't meant to win. It's time to put the weapons down.

The Scale Is a Liar

It is 7:00 AM on a Tuesday. You wake up feeling like a champion. You've had a "perfect" 48 hours; you swapped the evening takeout for a home-cooked dal, hit your 10,000 steps, and even walked past the office cupcakes with the stoic resolve of a Zen monk. You walk toward the bathroom with the quiet confidence of a winner, expecting the digital numbers to flash a transformation so profound the scale might actually thank you for your service.

Then, the numbers stop blinking. You've gained 600 grams.

In that single heartbeat, your entire mood shifts. The morning sun feels less bright, your breakfast tastes like cardboard, and that annoying voice in your head, let's call him the "Inner Critic", starts whispering: "See? It doesn't matter what you do. You're genetically destined for this. Pass the paratha." But here is the radical truth you need to tattooed on your brain: That number has almost nothing to do with your progress. The scale isn't a judge; it's a primitive piece of hardware measuring your relationship with gravity. It is, quite frankly, the most lying, toxic, and unreliable narrator in your health journey.

Welcome to Chapter 4. Grab a ginger tea, sit comfortably, and let's dismantle the box that's been hijacking your happiness.

1. The Great Metric Deception: Why Gravity Isn't Health
2. We've been conditioned to believe in a 1:1 ratio of Input to Output. We treat our bodies like a bank account: deposit a salad, withdraw a pound. But biology isn't a linear spreadsheet; it's a complex, beautiful, and sometimes moody ecosystem.

When you step on a scale, you aren't measuring your "worth," your "discipline," or even necessarily your fat. You are measuring a shifting cocktail of:

Bone density and organ weight (hopefully staying put!)

Undigested food (that high-fibre dinner is still "checking out")

Glycogen stores: For every gram of carbohydrate stored in your muscles for energy, your body holds onto about three to four grams of water.

The "Salt Spike": Had a slightly salty soup last night? Your body is currently holding onto water like a desert traveller, balancing those electrolytes.

The scale is like a "Mean Boss" who refuses to give you a raise even when you've worked overtime. It ignores the most important factor: body composition. I've seen my friends who look completely different; tighter, leaner, more vibrant; yet the scale hasn't moved an inch. Why? Because they've traded "fluff" for "firm."

1. Cotton vs. Iron: The Volume Paradox
2. To understand why the scale is a liar, we have to talk about the "Cotton vs. Iron" paradox.

If you have 1kg of cotton and 1kg of iron, which one is heavier? Neither; they both weigh exactly 1kg. But they look entirely different. The cotton is massive, fluffy, and takes up a huge amount of space. The iron is small, dense, and compact.

In your body, fat is the cotton; muscle is the iron. Muscle is significantly denser than fat. This means a kilogram of muscle takes up about 15-20% less space than a kilogram of fat. You can lose several inches off your waistline, your clothes can start to glide over your hips without "The Jump and Wiggle," and yet the scale might stay the same, or even go up.

If you are eating right and moving well, your body is moving toward "iron." The scale, being a blunt instrument, can't tell the difference. It just sees "mass." It doesn't know that the mass it's measuring is now high-quality, metabolic-boosting muscle rather than inflammatory fat.

1. The Science of the "False Increase" (The Post-Workout Trap)

2. This is where most people quit. You decide to get serious. You hit the gym on Monday and Tuesday. You're sore, you're tired, but you're proud. You step on the scale Wednesday morning and; boom; you're up a kilo.

   To the uneducated eye, this looks like failure. In reality, it is a biological "Congratulations."

   When you exercise, especially if you're lifting weights or trying a new HIIT class, you create microscopic tears in your muscle fibres. This isn't damage; it's the stimulus for growth. To repair those tears, your body initiates an inflammatory response. It sends fluid, white blood cells, and nutrients to the area to patch things up.

   This temporary water retention (oedema) shows up on the scale as weight gain. If you don't understand this, you might conclude that "exercise makes me fat" and punish yourself by working out even harder or cutting more calories. This increases stress, which raises cortisol, which, you guessed it, causes more water retention. It's a cycle of self-punishment fueled by a lack of physiological literacy.

1. Why Numbers Hijack the Heart: The "Waiting Room" Mentality

2. Why do we let a plastic box on the bathroom floor decide if we are allowed to be happy today? Because we've turned weight into a moral verdict. I remember a colleague, Meera. She was doing brilliantly. Her skin was glowing, her digestion had finally settled after years of bloating, and she was sleeping like a baby. But one morning, the scale showed a 300g increase. She called me in tears, ready to cancel her weekend plans. She felt she "hadn't earned" the right to go out.

   This is what I call the "Waiting Room of Life." We tell ourselves:

   "I'll wear that red dress when I'm 5kg lighter."

   "I'll apply for that promotion when I look the part."

   "I'll take the kids swimming when I've 'fixed' my thighs."

   We treat happiness like a luxury we haven't earned yet, convinced we must pay a "toll" in pounds before we deserve to participate in our own lives. But your value is not a variable that fluctuates with Earth's gravitational pull. You are not a "Before" picture waiting to become an "After." You are the main character of your life right now.

The "Root Cause" Check

If the scale is up, stop looking at the number and start looking at your Lifestyle Pillars. Ask yourself:

How was my sleep? (Poor sleep = High Cortisol = Water Retention).

How is my digestion? (Constipation can easily add 1-2kg of "weight" on a scale).

What was my stress level? (Stress makes the body hold on for dear life).

Am I hydrated? (Ironically, when you don't drink enough water, your body hoards what it has.)

Fix the root, and the fruit (the results) will follow. But the scale is the last thing to know the truth.

1. The "Ideal Weight" Myth: Who Defined Yours?
2. There is no such thing as a "generic" ideal weight. The BMI charts on your doctor's wall were created in the 1830s by a Belgian mathematician (not a doctor!) to measure populations, not individuals. They don't know your bone structure, your ethnic heritage, your muscle mass, or your soul.

The real "Ideal Weight" for you is the Weight of Well-being. It is the weight at which you are:

Active: You can climb a flight of stairs or play with your dog without gasping.

Pain-free: Your joints feel supported, and your inflammation is low.

Happy: You can enjoy a meal with your family without an internal calculator running in your head.

Stress-free: Your identity is no longer tied to a digital readout.

For some, their ideal weight might be 5kg heavier than the "chart" says, but at that weight, they have a menstrual cycle, thick hair, a high libido, and mental peace. Which one is "healthier"?

1. Relatability Check: The "Jeans Test"

2. If you want to measure progress, throw the scale in the attic and use the "Jeans Test." Find a pair of non-stretch denim. Try them on once every two weeks. Denim doesn't care about your water retention or your glycogen stores. Denim doesn't lie. If the jeans feel looser but your weight stays the same,

you are successfully changing your body composition. You are becoming "Iron."

3. Education is Empowerment: Don't Punish the Effort

4. The most heartbreaking thing I see is someone who has been "correct" all along, eating whole foods, sleeping well, moving their body, but gives up because of a "random" number.

When you see an increased number, do not conclude with incomplete knowledge. Do not assume you've failed. Do not punish yourself with an extra hour of cardio. Instead, stay the course. Consistency is the only thing that beats the scale's fluctuations. Results are often "latent"; they occur inside your cells, in your mitochondria, and in your gut microbiome, long before they appear in a 2D format on a scale.

Did You Know?

Your weight on the Moon would be about 16% of what it is on Earth. You wouldn't be "healthier" or "thinner" on the Moon; you'd just have less gravitational pull. If you're letting a number define your worth, remember that you're essentially letting your distance from the Earth's core determine your self-esteem. Seems a bit silly when you put it that way, doesn't it?

The Scale as a Bad Boyfriend

Think of the scale as a toxic partner. One day, he tells you you're amazing (low number), the next day, he's cold and distant and tells you you're a failure (high number). He doesn't know your heart, he doesn't care about your effort, and he's constantly gaslighting you.

Would you keep that person in your house? Probably not. At the very least, you'd stop taking his opinion seriously.

Reflection: The 15-Second "Non-Scale" Victory Check

Close your eyes. Forget the morning's weigh-in. Ask yourself:

Energy: How do I feel right now? Am I fueled or am I dragging?

Mood: Am I more patient today? More present?

Strength: Did I lift something today that felt heavy last month?

Conclusion: Don't let numbers hijack your happiness. Life is a happy journey, and some random digits on a bathroom floor cannot; and will not; become the mission of your life. Your body is a vessel for your soul, not a math problem to be solved. Be patient. Be consistent. Be kind.

The scale is a liar. You, however, are the truth.

The Shame Nobody Sees

If chronic dieting is the war, then shame is the invisible shrapnel that stays lodged in your skin long after the battle is over. We've spent the previous chapters talking about the scale and the mind, but now we need to talk about the *world.* Because you don't live in a vacuum. You live in a world where your body is often treated like public property; a landscape that everyone from your boss to the distant aunt at a family wedding feel entitled to "zone," critique, and "fix."

This is the shame nobody sees because we've been taught to carry it quietly, like a heavy suitcase we aren't allowed to put down. It is the specific pain of judgment replacing empathy, and the societal "eye-roll" that greets anyone living in a larger body. It's a weight that doesn't show up on the scale, but it's heavy enough to crush your spirit before you even step out of the house.

The "Entitled" Observer: Home, Work, and Society

We've all experienced it. You haven't seen a particular relative in six months, and before they even say "Hello" or ask how your career is going, their eyes do a quick, predatory sweep of your torso.

"Beta, you've filled out! Are you eating too much rice?" It is delivered with a smile, but it lands like a physical blow to the stomach. In our society, body shaming is frequently disguised as "concern." At home, it's the parent who stares at your plate during dinner, silently counting your rotis. At work, it's the colleague who makes a "joke" about the office snacks while looking pointedly at you.

I remember a time when I had finally, with Herculean effort and immense self-control, managed to lose some weight. I was glowing. I felt like I had finally cracked the code, and for the first time in years, I felt a sense of pride in my discipline. But instead of people celebrating my vitality, I noticed a strange, dark shift in the attention I received. The whispers changed. The interpretation from those around me wasn't that I was getting healthy; it was that I must be depressed.

Suddenly, I was receiving "pity care." People were extra gentle, asking if I was "okay" with a tilted head and a sad pout. The assumption was that if a woman like me loses weight, she must be going through a tragedy. It felt like a "no-win" game: if I was heavier, I was "lazy"; if I was thinner, I was "broken." Why is it so hard for society to see a person's health journey as an act of power rather than a symptom of a problem?

The Humiliation of the "Public Eye"

The public sphere isn't much kinder. There is a specific kind of trauma that happens in shared spaces when you feel your body takes up "too much" room.

I remember travelling by public transport, minding my own business, when someone would stand up and offer me a seat with a knowing, sympathetic smile. For a long time, I took it as a random act of kindness; the kind of "humanity still exists" moment you'd post about. It wasn't until a friend pointed out the brutal, humiliating truth: *"They think you're pregnant because of your belly."* I wasn't even married. In that moment, the bus felt like it had shrunk to the size of a matchbox. I wanted the floor to open up. It is a perfect example of how being overweight is construed as an "illness" or a "condition" by the public. Total strangers feel they have the right to diagnose you, pity you, or accommodate you based on a silhouette they don't understand. This isn't just an "awkward moment"; it's Weight Bias, and research shows it can be as psychologically damaging as other forms of discrimination, leading to higher levels of cortisol and, ironically, further weight gain due to stress.

Judgment Replacing Empathy

The biggest lie society tells is that being overweight is a simple choice. This narrative, supported by a billion-dollar fitness industry, suggests that if you just "wanted it enough," you'd be thin.

But no one understands that nobody *chooses* the struggle. Nobody chooses the joint pain, the breathless climb up the stairs, or the wardrobe filled with "hiding clothes." Yet, everyone is ready to give you a piece of their mind. Your uncle has a "magic keto trick," your friend has a "secret herbal tea," and your Instagram feed is a toxic slurry of influencers telling you to "grind harder."

What they lack is empathy. They don't see the biological uphill battle; the hormones like ghrelin (the hunger hormone) that skyrocket when you diet, or the leptin resistance that makes your brain think you're starving even when you've just eaten. Research in social psychology shows that weight bias is one of the last socially acceptable forms of prejudice. They see a "problem" to be solved, rather than a human being to be supported.

The "Concerned" Colleague

The setting: The office cafeteria. You've brought a balanced, healthy meal. The Scenario: A colleague watches you eat and says, *"Oh, you're being so good today! I saw you had pizza at the team lunch on Friday, though. Is this your 'reset'?* "The Impact: Suddenly, your meal is no longer about nourishment; it's a performance. You feel the heat of shame rising because your food choices are being "tracked" by a third party. The Truth: This isn't support; it's surveillance. Support looks like talking about your weekend, your projects, or your dreams; not the contents of your Tupperware.

The "Rehab" of the Mind

Let's reframe this. Losing weight is easy when it is teamwork. We often look at the word "Rehabilitation" with a negative lens, associating it with rock bottom or "brokenness." But think about what a rehab setup actually is: it's a controlled environment filled with guidance, nutritional support, and, most importantly, mental fitness.

The day we start asking for help, true, empathetic help, it becomes simpler. Asking for help isn't a sign of weakness; it's an admission that the mountain is high and we'd prefer a climbing partner. Getting fit is a massive challenge. Some people are "blessed" with high metabolisms or were raised in environments where they were never made to feel small, and thus, they are unaware of the struggle. We can't change their luck.

But we should thank God for our awareness. We have the courage to address an issue and accept it willingly. We should be incredibly proud of ourselves. We are the ones who aren't waiting for a "medical alarm" through a scary lab report or a doctor's grim face to start. We are taking the initiative because we know we need to be healthy for *ourselves*, not for the "aunty" or the "bus passenger."

The Biological Cost of Shame

Psychologically, shame is a "secondary emotion." It usually hides a more profound need for safety and belonging. When we are shamed by society, our nervous system enters a state of "threat."

When you feel judged, your brain's amygdala triggers the "fight or flight" response. This increases cortisol, which tells your body to store fat (especially around the abdomen) to prepare for a perceived emergency. So, in a cruel twist of irony, the people shaming you "for your own health" are actually creating the exact biological environment that prevents health. Empathy, on the other hand, lowers stress and allows the body to move into a state of "rest and digest." Support is literally medicine.

We must move from a place of *"I hate my body, so I must change it"* to *"I love my life, so I must support my body."* When you accept that your body is currently doing the best it can to protect you, the external comments start to lose their sting. You realise that their judgment is a reflection of *their* limited mindsets, not *your* worth. You are a warrior because you have the awareness to face a challenge that others ignore.

Pause & Notice

Before you close this chapter, I want you to sit in a quiet space for 30 seconds. Think about the last time you were harsh to yourself; perhaps it was after a meal or after seeing your reflection in a shop window. Now, ask yourself:

"Would I speak to a dear friend this way?"

If a friend came to you crying because they felt humiliated on public transport or judged at a family dinner, would you tell them they were "lazy"? Would you tell them they don't deserve a seat? Of course not. You would hug them. You would say to them they are brave for showing up in a world that doesn't always make room for them. You would tell them that their belly is just a small part of a magnificent, complex person.

You deserve the same empathy you give so freely to others. You are not a "Before" picture waiting to happen; you are a whole human being deserving of respect right now. The "Shame Nobody Sees" only has power as long as we keep it a secret. Once we voice it, once we acknowledge it, and once we demand empathy over judgment, its power begins to fade.

You are not waiting for an alarm. You are already awake. And that, in itself, is a victory.

Reflections for the Soul:

- *Who are the people in my life who make me feel "safe" regardless of my size?*
- *What boundaries do I need to set with the "Aunties" (at home or work) to protect my peace?*
- *Can I acknowledge my courage today?*

PART II: THE ADDICTION & THE INDUSTRY

Instant Results & the Dopamine Trap

By this point in our lives, many of us have "arrived." We've climbed the corporate ladder, built businesses, or navigated the complexities of adulting with a fair amount of grace. We are successful, we are confident, and fortunately, we finally have the financial muscle to buy the things we want. In every other area of life, if a pipe bursts, we hire the best plumber. If our car breaks down, we pay for the premium service. We are used to paying for solutions and seeing immediate results.

But then, we look in the mirror.

Our body remains the one area where our professional success and our bank balance don't seem to hold any sway. It feels like a nagging "unfinished project." And because we are busy, high-achieving people, we apply our professional logic to our physical health: We try to buy a shortcut. We look for the most expensive, most exclusive "quick fix" available. There's a psychological hook here; we've been conditioned to believe that if something is cheap, it's fake; if it's expensive, it must be "medical grade" or "elite." We throw money at the problem to stroke our ego and silence the body that keeps reminding us of the one thing we haven't mastered.

Welcome to the world of the Dopamine Trap.

1. The High-Price Shortcut: Buying the Illusion

When you're successful, you don't want a "slow and steady" walk. You want a rocket ship. We fall for the tempting offers: the 10-day "liquid gold" detox retreats, the imported meal-replacement shakes that cost more than a fine dining experience in Dubai, or the "VIP Keto" plans that promise a new you by next Sunday.

For a moment, it works. You spend the money, you follow the grueling, restrictive hacks, and the scale actually moves. You see Instant Results. Your ego gets a massive boost. You walk into the office feeling as if you've finally conquered the final frontier. People start to notice. The compliments roll in like a flood of digital dopamine: *"Wow, you look amazing! What's the secret?"*

Deep down, in the quiet moments before sleep, a small voice whispers the truth: *This is temporary.* You know you cannot live on liquid shakes or zero-carb plates for the rest of your life. You know you're living on borrowed time. But the dopamine high is so intoxicating that you choose to live in denial. You've arrived, or so you tell yourself.

2. The Dopamine High vs. The Emotional Crash

In the world of brain chemistry, dopamine is the "reward" molecule. It's the rush you get when you see a lower number on the scale or get a "like" on a transformation photo. But dopamine has a dark twin: The Crash.

Crash diets and shortcuts are essentially "biochemical credit cards." You are spending energy and health today that you haven't actually earned, and eventually, the bill comes due.

- The High: Week 1-3. You feel invincible. You're losing 2kg a week. You're "winning."
- The Plateau: Week 4. The body realises it's being starved. It enters "Survival Mode," slowing down your thyroid and cranking up your hunger hormones.
- The Crash: Week 6. Cravings turn into obsessions. Fatigue seeps into your bones. Frustration replaces pride.

When you inevitably "get off" the diet, because your sister is getting married or you just couldn't face another day of cabbage soup, the weight doesn't just return; it rushes back with interest. This is where the situation becomes severe. Because you used a shortcut, you never learned how to actually walk the path. When the results vanish, you don't just feel "heavy"; you feel depressed. The emotional balance is gone. Because you tied your success to a "hack," your failure feels like a character flaw. You lose the ability to look at your health neutrally. You fall into a dark pit of sadness, convinced that if the "best, most expensive" plan didn't work, nothing will.

3. The biology of the "Bounce Back"

Let's look at the numbers the industry tries to hide. Research from UCLA suggests that up to two-thirds of people who lose weight on restrictive diets end up gaining back *more* than they lost within four or five years. Why? Because of a biological phenomenon called Adaptive Thermogenesis. When you slash your calories or cut out entire food groups, your body doesn't think, "Oh, we're trying to look good for the beach!" It thinks, "We are in a famine. Shut down the power plants." Your metabolic rate drops. Your body becomes more efficient at storing fat.

So, when you finally eat a regular meal again, your "thrifty" metabolism grabs every single calorie and shoves it into storage. You aren't failing because you lack willpower; you are failing because you are fighting a million years of human evolution. You cannot out-willpower your DNA.

4. The Ego and the "Expert"

Our ego tells us, *"I'm a leader, I can handle a 20-hour fast."* Our body says, *"I'm a biological organism, and I'm stressed out."*

The most "elite" thing you can do for your health isn't buying an expensive supplement; it's finding the right teachers. We need to educate ourselves and learn from people who understand the long game. For example, did you know that most "detox" shakes actually slow down your liver's natural Phase II detoxification because they lack the necessary amino acids found in real food? You are paying **$200** to make your liver less efficient; in India, the same detox fantasy is repackaged as influencer-led cleanse programs and overpriced powders sold at a steep premium to common sense. That's not a hack; that's a scam.

Success in health looks like:

- Nuance over Noise: Understanding that "One size fits all" fits nobody.

- Neutrality over Emotion: Seeing a weight fluctuation as "data," not a "disaster."
- Consistency over Intensity: Realising that a 20-minute walk every day for a year is infinitely more potent than a 3-hour gym session that leaves you injured and exhausted.

Myth vs. Reality

The Myth: Fast results are the only way to stay motivated.

The Reality: Fast results are often "water weight" and muscle loss. Losing muscle is the worst thing you can do for your long-term weight management, as muscle is your primary calorie-burning engine. Research shows that "Rapid Weight Loss" (more than 1.5kg per week) can trigger a permanent drop in metabolic rate. Slow progress is the only progress that sticks.

5. The "Rent vs. Own" Model

Think of a crash diet like renting a luxury apartment. You look great while you're in it, but the moment you stop paying the "rent" (the extreme restriction), you're evicted. You have no equity. You own nothing.

Sustainable health is about Home Ownership. It takes longer to save the down payment. It's a lot of tedious paperwork (education). But once you own the "home", once you understand how your gut microbiome works, how sleep affects insulin, and how to eat for your specific body, nobody can evict you. You carry the "home" of health with you everywhere you go.

6. The Cost of Denial

We often live in denial while we're on these shortcuts. We ignore the hair thinning, the brittle nails, the irritability, and the loss of libido. We tell ourselves it's "worth it" because the scale is moving. But what is the point of being a size smaller if you are too tired to enjoy the clothes you're wearing?

This is the Dopamine Trap in its purest form: choosing a short-term hit of validation over a long-term state of vitality. We trade our peace of mind for a temporary pat on the back.

7. Reclaiming Your Power

You cannot buy a fit body, but you can invest in the awareness required to create one. The "Shortcut" is the longest path because it's a circle; it always brings you back to where you started, but with more baggage and less confidence.

It's time to stop trying to "control" the outcome and start "nurturing" the organism. You've worked hard for your money and your career. Don't let a "Dopamine Trap" steal the one thing money can't buy: a peaceful, sustainable relationship with your own body.

15-Second Awareness Pause

Put down this book. Take one deep, intentional breath. Feel the air enter your lungs and exit your body. Now, ask yourself:

1. The "Why": Am I looking for a "New Me," or am I just looking for a "Quick Escape" from the "Old Me"?

2. The "Sustainability": If I had to do what I'm doing today every day for the next three years, would I be happy or miserable?

3. The "Truth": Am I spending money to avoid the hard work of actually getting to know my body?

If the answer is "Quick Escape" or "Miserable," it's okay. You aren't failing; you're just trapped in a loop designed to keep you spending. The exit is right here. It starts with the decision to stop rushing.

Weight Loss as an Addiction

I remember a colleague of mine, Maya. She was a powerhouse, a top-tier executive who could navigate a boardroom with the precision of a chess grandmaster. She came to see me after a gruelling 12-week "Extreme Transformation" program she'd bought from a flashy influencer for a price that could have funded a small island. She had lost fifteen kilograms. By every societal metric, she had "arrived." Her cheekbones were sculpted, her waist was tiny, and she was fitting into the kind of high-fashion silhouettes she hadn't touched in a decade.

But as she sat in our office, she wasn't celebrating. She was trembling. "I'm terrified," she whispered, her voice cracking. "I'm terrified of a slice of sourdough. I'm terrified of waking up and seeing the scale move by even a hundred grams. I feel like if I'm not losing, I'm failing. If I'm not shrinking, I'm disappearing."

Maya wasn't just a dieter anymore. She had developed an addiction. Not to a substance, but to the "Thin High." She was chasing the ecstatic rush of the drop, and like any person with an addiction, she was one "fix" away from a total emotional and physiological collapse.

The Ecstasy of the Drop

When you first taste success on a radical weight-loss plan, the feeling is intoxicating. It's a rush that rivals any chemical stimulant. Suddenly, the world looks different. People smile at you more. You feel lighter, faster, and more powerful. This is the "honeymoon phase" of weight loss, where your brain is flooded with dopamine, the neurotransmitter of reward and anticipation. You've finally "cracked the code," and you want to stay in that high forever.

But here is the catch: because those results were often achieved through "wrong means", extreme restriction, metabolic manipulation, or unsustainable hacks, the high is inherently fragile. Your body is a biological machine, not a digital avatar. It cannot sustain a state of emergency indefinitely. When the results inevitably stall, or the weight starts to creep back, the reaction is almost identical to a drug addict going through withdrawal. You feel a loss of motivation, a sudden surge of aggressive anger, and an irritability that makes you want to snap at a cloud for being too fluffy.

The Biochemistry of the Craving

To understand why Maya felt like a person with an addiction, we have to look at what's happening under the hood. This isn't about "weakness"; it's about a survival mechanism that has been fine-tuned over millions of years. When you lose weight rapidly, your body thinks you are trapped in a famine.

Two key hormones go into battle: Leptin and Ghrelin. Think of Leptin as the "Fuel Gauge" (it tells the brain you have enough fat stored) and Ghrelin as the "Grumbling Belly" (it screams for food). In a crash diet, your Fuel Gauge breaks (Leptin drops) and your Grumbling Belly turns into a megaphone (Ghrelin spikes).

Your brain enters a state of "Homeostatic Hunger",; which is basically a fancy way of saying your body's internal thermostat is set to "Starving." It begins to hyper-sensitise your reward system. Suddenly, a commercial for a burger isn't just an ad; it's a siren song. Your brain increases the dopamine response to high-calorie foods, making the "craving" feel like a life-or-death necessity. You aren't just "hungry"; your brain is demanding a chemical fix to restore the energy it thinks you've lost. It's why you can find yourself at 11 PM staring into the fridge like it's a holy relic, contemplating if frozen peas count as a snack.

Family & Friends

This is the part we often underplay. When we are chasing the "high" of weight loss or crashing from the "low" of regain, we don't suffer alone. Our emotions become dependent on unreasonable and impossible results, and when the scale doesn't cooperate, our family and friends get the brunt of our depression.

Imagine a dinner table moment: Your spouse has spent an hour cooking a beautiful meal. Instead of enjoying the company, you are sitting there, eyes darting, mentally calculating the "caloric debt" of the gravy. When they ask you to take a bite, you don't see love; you see a threat to your progress. You snap. You get angry. The mood in the room dies instantly.

Or think about the missed birthdays. You skip your best friend's celebration because you're "not in your goal size" and you can't face the judgment you *imagine* everyone has. You have a work meltdown because the brain fog from your zero-carb lunch means you can't remember the password to your own presentation. These mood swings affect your daily routines, your core responsibilities, and your relationships. It is a cascading effect; one "bad" number on the scale on Tuesday leads to a fight with your partner on Wednesday and a missed deadline on Thursday. You are living in a state of irrationality, not realising that these are actions you will surely regret when you finally understand the reality.

The Industry of Vulnerability

The cruel world of commerce knows exactly how you feel. They count on your vulnerability. This is where the "New Invention" cycle begins. Just as you are hitting your lowest point of withdrawal, a new advertisement appears on your feed, promising a "breakthrough" or a "secret ice hack." These fake promises look incredibly real because you are in a state of Cognitive Dissonance; that mental tug-of-war where you *know* the last diet failed you, but you *want* to believe this new one is the "One." It's like texting an ex-boyfriend you know is evil for you because you're lonely. The industry doesn't want to cure you; it wants to keep you in the cycle of "Search, Buy, Fail, Repeat." If you actually got healthy and stayed that way, you'd stop being a recurring revenue stream.

The Business of Failure

- 80–95% Failure Rate: Peer-reviewed studies consistently show that 80–95% of diets fail long-term. Most people regain the weight within 2 to 5 years.

- Recession-Proof Growth: The weight loss industry thrives on repeated failure. It is valued at over $250 billion globally (which translates to a multi-lakh-crore industry in India alone). Your "failure" is literally their business model. They sell the "hope" of the fix, knowing the biology is rigged against the method.

Moving Toward Rationality

To move past this addiction, we have to become practical. We have to stop expecting the "impossible" and start understanding the "biological." In the world of top-tier wellness experts like Luke Coutinho or Ritesh Bawri, the focus is on Mental Fitness. You cannot have physical health without a stable, rational mind.

Health isn't a "drop" on a scale; it's a state of internal harmony. You have to realise that:

- Your body is not your enemy: It is a brilliant organism trying to protect you.
- Shortcuts are detours: Every "quick fix" adds another layer of trauma to your metabolism.
- Addiction thrives in the "all or nothing": A healthy person thinks in averages. If you have a meal that wasn't "on plan," a

rational person says, "That was delicious," and moves on. A person with a substance use disorder says, "The day is ruined, I'm a failure," and orders the entire dessert menu.

The "Rehab" of the Soul

We need to look at the term "rehabilitation" with pride. Asking for help is the simplest way to shorten the road. When you seek guidance from those who prioritise food as medicine and mental resilience, the journey becomes a team effort.

Some people are "blessed" with unawareness; they never had to fight this battle. But you? You have awareness. You have the courage to address the issue and accept it willingly. You aren't waiting for the "alarm" of a medical report or a lifestyle disease to start. You are taking the initiative because you respect your life. That makes you a leader, not a victim.

Hunger vs. Emotion Test

The next time you feel an overwhelming urge to eat something specific, take 60 seconds to play this game.

1. The "Boring Food" Test: If I offered you a plain bowl of dal or a hard-boiled egg right now, would you eat it?

- *Yes?* You are physically hungry.

- *No, I only want that specific samosa?* You are chasing a dopamine fix.

2. The "Suddenness" Check: Did this hunger grow slowly over the last two hours, or did it hit you the second your boss sent a "Can we talk?" email?

- *Gradual?* Physical.
- *Sudden?* Emotional.

3. The "Body Scan": Is your stomach growling, or is your mind just "looping" on a specific texture?

- *Stomach?* Physical.
- *Head/Mouth?* Emotional.

The Insight: If it's emotional, the food will never be enough. You are hungry for a feeling: safety or comfort. Address the feeling, not the plate.

The Homecoming

Remember Maya? We didn't prescribe a new diet or tell her what to eat. We focused on mental fitness together until she realised her worth wasn't tied to her dress size. She moved away from chasing the "Thin High" and toward the "Vitality

Glow", that steady, calm energy that comes from nourishing the body, not punishing it.

Don't let the industry hijack your dopamine. Don't let a temporary "high" cost you your relationships or your peace. You are worth more than a number. Weight loss shouldn't feel like an addiction; it should feel like a homecoming. It's time to stop chasing the "drop" and start embracing the life you've been putting on hold. You already have the awareness, you have the courage, and now, you have the truth.

Sold Stories, Bought Shame

I recently found myself in the digital equivalent of a dark alley: scrolling through Instagram at 2:00 AM while the rest of Mumbai slept. I stopped at a reel of a woman who looked like Renaissance masters had sculpted her and then airbrushed by a supercomputer, glowing under ring lights that made her look like a Bollywood starlet off-duty. She was radiant, tossing organic blueberries and expensive Amla into a high-end blender, her smile suggesting she had never known a day of bloating after a heavy wedding biryani. The caption read: "How I lost 15kg in 30 days drinking this morning elixir! Click the link in my bio for my $99 'Glow-Up' protocol." Even though the price was set in USD, my mind instantly did the frantic math, realizing that for an Indian household, this "magical" liquid was costing roughly 8,300 rupees; more than a month's worth of high-quality groceries or a premium gym membership; yet the lure of the quick fix felt so potent that the $99 seemed like a small ransom to pay for the dream body we are conditioned to chase.

Even with my education, my professional background, and my deep understanding of the health industry's smoke and mirrors, I felt it, that familiar, insidious tug. My heart raced. A desperate, irrational voice in my head whispered, *"What if?*

What if she actually has the secret? What if I'm just one $99 payment away from never worrying about my body again?" This is the "Trade-off Deal" we offer ourselves in the quiet hours: we are willing to risk our hard-earned money and our sanity for the chance, however slim, of gaining our dream body. Our gut warns us; it screams that this is a waste of effort. Yet, we silence it. We want to believe we are "The Lucky One." We aren't just buying a PDF; we are buying a story. And unfortunately, the stories being sold are often built on a foundation of lies, lighting, and a dangerous psychological phenomenon called Survivorship Bias.

1. The Architecture of the Digital Illusion

Social media is not a window; it is a meticulously curated stage. Before that influencer hit "record" on her "What I Eat in a Day" video, a massive amount of invisible labour took place to ensure you felt just enough shame to reach for your credit card.

The Invisible Sculptors

First, let's talk about Lighting Tricks. High-angle, soft lighting can instantly erase cellulite and shadows. Professional fitness photographers use "down-lighting" to create artificial muscle definition that disappears the moment you walk into a room with a standard ceiling bulb. Then comes the Posing. There is a specific way to tilt the pelvis, hold the breath, and engage the core, often called "vacuuming", that makes the stomach look concave. It's an athletic feat to hold that pose for the three seconds it takes to snap the photo.

The AI and Filter Frontier

We are now in an era where "Real-Time Body Filters" can slim a waistline even in a moving video. You aren't competing with a fit person; you are competing with a digital hallucination. When you see a "What I Eat in a Day" video where a creator eats half an avocado and three almonds but has the energy of a marathon runner, you are seeing an illusion. Research shows that many of these creators struggle with disordered eating or simply don't film the other 70% of what they actually consume. They sell you the 30-second highlight reel, and you buy it with your self-esteem.

2. Why the "Lucky One" Isn't a Metric

This is a concept used by top-tier wellness experts to explain why generic advice is often "biological garbage." Survivorship Bias is the logical error of focusing on the people who "made it" through a specific process and ignoring those who didn't; mainly because the "failures" are silent.

Imagine 1,000 people try a dangerous "Cabbage Soup and Caffeine" diet:

- Nine hundred ninety people end up with hair loss, ruined metabolisms, and eventual weight regain. They don't post about it because they feel embarrassed and "weak."
- Ten people have a specific genetic makeup that allows them to survive the restriction without their thyroid shutting down.
- 1 of those 10 becomes an influencer and sells the plan as a "proven system."

You see one success and conclude: *"If it worked for her, it must work for me."* You don't see the 990 "biological bodies" left in the wake of that diet. You think you're buying a map, but you're actually buying a lottery ticket where the odds are stacked against your DNA.

3. The "Ratatouille" Rule

In the movie *Ratatouille*, Chef Gusteau famously says, *"Anyone can cook."* It's a beautiful, inclusive sentiment. However, in the world of health, we must add a cynical footnote: "Anyone can lose weight, but not everyone should teach you how."

Just because someone has a six-pack doesn't mean they understand human physiology, endocrinology, or gut health. Many influencers are "Genetically Blessed" or "Metabolically Young." They have high metabolic flexibility, allowing them to bounce back from any stupidity they put their bodies through. When they tell you to "just stop eating carbs," they aren't giving you a health protocol; they are giving you their personal autobiography.

A world-class nutritionist understands Bio-Individuality. What heals one person might be "metabolic poison" to another. For example, a high-fat Keto diet might help a sedentary person with insulin resistance, but it could wreck the hormones of a high-stress executive with adrenal fatigue. When we buy "Sold Stories," we are ignoring our own unique biological signature.

Myth vs. Reality

The Myth: If a plan worked for a celebrity or a viral influencer, it is a scientifically valid path for my body.

The Reality: Success in weight loss is often a "Perfect Storm" of genetics, age, sleep quality, and history. Following someone else's plan is like wearing someone else’s prescription glasses;

it might look stylish on the outside, but you'll end up with a massive headache and blurred vision on the inside.

4. Vulnerability as a Business Model

The social media giants and AI algorithms are at their most efficient when we are at our most vulnerable. They track our searches. If you've looked up "how to hide a bloated stomach" at 2:00 AM, the algorithm marks you as "Desperate." It starts feeding you "Rosy Results." It plays on the "Trade-off Deal" our brain makes: *"I'll spend 5,000 rupees now if it means I don't have to feel this shame anymore."* Sensibly, it is a waste of money, but the lure of the "Quick Fix" acts like a chemical drug. This is Predatory Marketing. It doesn't sell health; it sells a temporary escape from the "Bought Shame" they helped manufacture. They make you feel bad about your body, then sell you the "cure" for the very feeling they created. It's a brilliant, cruel circle of commerce.

5. Educating the Gut

How do we stop getting fooled? We have to move from being "Consumers" to being "Stewards." We need to look for the Red Flags in the stories we are sold:

- The "One Ingredient" Miracle: If they say one "magic berry" or "ice hack" does all the work, they are lying.
- The "Short Timeline": Anything promising permanent change in 30 days ignores how human cells actually regenerate.
- The "Vibe over Science": If the post focuses more on the creator's bikini than on the biology of the gut-brain axis, keep scrolling.

Authentic health is inherently "boring" because it lacks the high-octane drama of a viral reel, favouring the quiet consistency of eating local, seasonal foods like a comforting plate of *Dal Chawal* paired with a side of home-made fermented pickles. While the global wellness industry tries to sell us on the latest trends, it is startling to realise that a single, humble piece of *Amla* (Indian Gooseberry), which costs barely ₹5 to ₹10 at your local street vendor, provides a far more potent and bioavailable dose of Vitamin C than a flashy $50 synthetic gummy endorsed by a celebrity. Even without converting that dollar price into rupees, the sheer absurdity of spending such a staggering amount on a processed supplement highlights the "Bought Shame" culture we've fallen into; in the Indian context, that same $50 (roughly ₹4,200) could fund a family's entire stock of fresh, organic vegetables and seasonal fruits for nearly a month. We often ignore the goldmine of nutrition in our own backyards to chase expensive, imported labels, forgetting that true vitality isn't found in a premium bottle, but in the sunshine on our skin, eight hours of deep sleep, and the time-tested wisdom of our traditional kitchens.

6. The Science of the "Un-glamorous"

To show the extent of research required to truly heal, consider the Circadian Rhythm of Food. Top wellness experts now know that *when* you eat is often as important as *what* you eat. Your body's ability to process glucose is significantly higher in the morning than at night.

Instead of a "shimmering elixir," try these research-backed, un-glamorous options:

- Sequential Eating: Eating your fibre (salad) first, then protein, and finally carbs can blunt your blood sugar spike by up to 75%.
- The 10-Minute Walk: A short walk after a meal does more for your insulin sensitivity than almost any "fat-burning" supplement on the market.

- Probiotic Diversity: Homemade *Dahi* (curd) contains strains of bacteria that are specifically adapted to your local environment.

These aren't "hacks"; they are physiological principles. They don't cost $99, and they don't require a filter to work.

7. The 15-Second Feed Awareness Check

The next time you are scrolling and see a "Transformation Story" that makes your heart sink, pause for 15 seconds and run this filter:

1. The Environment: "Is this person tensing their muscles or using a beauty filter?"
2. The Logic: "Am I seeing the thousands of people this plan *didn't* work for?"
3. The Feeling: "Do I feel inspired to care for my body, or do I suddenly feel like I need to 'fix' it?"

The Rule: If a post makes you feel shame, unfollow it. Shame is the primary ingredient in the industry's profit margin.

Writing Your Own Story

We started this chapter with the lure of the "Lucky One." But the truth is, you don't need luck; you need loyalty to yourself. Don't let a digital avatar sell you a story that ignores your reality. You are a well-educated, modern person. You have the awareness to see the "Bought Shame" for what it is: a marketing tactic.

Your gut was right all along. The waste of money and effort isn't because you failed; it’s because the "deal" was rigged from the start. Stop buying other people's stories and start listening to your own body’s data. You aren't a "before" waiting for a "magic" after. You are the architect of your own vitality, and the most brilliant transformation isn't the one that happens on Instagram; it’s the one that occurs when you finally stop being fooled by the stories you were never meant to fit into.

Slow Cooking vs. The 10-Minute Recipe Myth

I remember visiting my grandmother's kitchen during monsoons, in a small town in Delhi, a sanctuary she had built after they had to migrate from the Sind province. The air was thick with the scent of damp earth and the hypnotic, slow-drifting aroma of burning coal from her *sigree*, the traditional iron stove that cradled the fire. Bebe sat on a low wooden stool, her hands moving with a meditative grace as she sorted through lentils. There were no flashing timers, no high-speed blenders, and indeed no "instant" settings. I, a city-bred youth fueled by the adrenaline of "productivity," once asked her, "Bebe, why do you soak the dal for four hours? And why does the subzi have to simmer for so long? I saw a video that says you can make Matar Paneer in ten minutes."

She looked at me with a smile that carried the wisdom of a thousand monsoons. "Beta," she said, "the fire softens the grain, but the time awakens its soul. If you rush the food, the food will rush through you, leaving nothing behind but a heavy heart and a bloated belly." Decades later, standing in a world obsessed with "10-minute healthy meal prep" and "instant air-fryer hacks," Bebe's words echo like a scientific prophecy. We have traded the soul of our food for the speed of our schedules. We have fallen for the 10-Minute Recipe Myth, forgetting that biology, unlike your internet connection, doesn't have a "fast-forward" button.

1. The Ancestral Flame: Cooking Before the Cylinder

To understand why slow cooking is a biological necessity, we have to look back long before the invention of gas cylinders or induction cooktops. Think of our ancestors in caves or the early civilizations that cooked on a *chulha*. There was no "high flame" dial. Cooking was an exercise in patience.

They used heavy clay pots or cast-iron vessels that retained heat. The fire was steady, low, and persistent. This slow application of heat did something magical: it allowed the food to undergo a deep chemical transformation. Complex starches were broken down into digestible sugars, and tough fibers were tenderized without being "shocked" into a rubbery state. This wasn't just about survival; it was the original "bio-hacking." Our bodies evolved to eat food that had been prepared with time.

2. The Instagram Illusion: The Danger of the 10-Minute "Miracle"

Fast-forward to today. Your Facebook feed or Instagram Explore page is a conveyor belt of "10-minute Matar Paneer" or "Instant Carrot Halwa." They show a blur of jump-cuts, a splash of oil, a toss of pre-cut frozen veggies, and *voila!* A glistening dish ready in seconds. But let's pull back the curtain on these "miracles." To make Matar Paneer in ten minutes, you usually have to bypass the most critical steps of Indian cooking:

- The Sauté (*Bhuna*): In a traditional kitchen, onions, ginger, and garlic are sautéed slowly until the raw sulfurous compounds are gone and the sugars caramelize. Rushing this leads to raw acidity that wreaks havoc on your gut lining.
- The Fibre Breakdown: A "10-minute" Gajar Halwa usually means the carrots haven't been cooked enough to break down the cellulose, or they've been drowned in condensed sugar to mask the raw taste.

When you eat these "shortcut" meals, you aren't just saving time; you are shifting the labour of cooking from the stove to your stomach. If digestion worked at Instagram speed, we wouldn't need stomachs. We'd just have a conveyor belt. Your gut has to produce extra acid and enzymes to deal with the "untransformed" food, leading to the "stone-in-the-stomach" feeling we've all grown accustomed to.

3. Traditional Indian Wisdom: The Science of Slowness

Traditional Indian cooking is a masterclass in Slow Chemistry. Our ancestors didn't have laboratories, but they had an intuitive understanding of bioavailability.

- Soaking: Why do we soak *Rajma* or *Chana* overnight? It's not just to make them soft. Soaking activates the enzyme *phytase*, which breaks down phytic acid. Phytic acid is an "anti-nutrient" that binds to minerals like iron and zinc, preventing your body from absorbing them. Without soaking, that "healthy" dal is actually stealing minerals from your body.

- Simmering: Slow cooking allows fat-soluble vitamins in spices (like the curcumin in turmeric) to fully infuse into the dish's fats. This makes the nutrients "bioavailable," meaning your cells can actually use them.

- Fermentation: Think of the *Idli* or *Dosa*. This is "pre-digestion" done by beneficial Bebecteria. It increases B-vitamins and makes the grain easier for the gut to digest.

4. Pressure Cooking: Efficiency Under Pressure

Now, let's talk about the modern Indian hero: the Pressure Cooker. While it feels "fast," the pressure cooker is actually a high-efficiency version of slow cooking. By sealing the environment, it uses pressure to raise the boiling point, cooking the food deeply and evenly without the nutrient loss associated with open-boiling or deep-frying.

According to the National Institute of Nutrition (2021), pressure cooking and steaming preserve up to 90% of Vitamin C. It effectively kills lectins, proteins in pulses that cause gut inflammation, making them much safer for your microbiome.

Did You Know?

Pressure cooking improves digestibility. By breaking down difficult-to-digest fibres and neutralizing lectins in pulses, the pressure cooker essentially does the "heavy lifting" for your stomach, significantly reducing post-meal gas and bloating.

5. Ultra-Processed Shortcut Culture: The Invisible Cost

The "10-minute" promise usually relies on "Ultra-Processed Shortcuts."

1. Pre-cooked packets: Loaded with preservatives and sodium to keep them shelf-stable.

2. Refined flour: Stripped of fibre to ensure it cooks in a blink.
3. Hidden sugars: Used to mimic the deep, caramelised flavour that only time can produce.

Speed has replaced process, and the cost is our resilience. When we choose the "2-minute" noodle over the "20-minute" khichdi, we aren't just saving 18 minutes; we are incurring a biological debt. The consequences are visible everywhere: early fatigue, weak bones, and persistent joint pain.

6. Eating Speed: The Final Frontier

It isn't just about how we cook; it's about how we consume. Slow-cooked food inherently invites slower eating. It has texture, aroma, and a complexity that demands attention. Ultra-soft, ultra-processed food is designed to be inhaled. Research shows that eating slowly increases levels of satiety hormones; your brain finally gets the memo that you are full. You cannot rush digestion without consequences. When you rush the cooking, you usually rush the eating, and your metabolic health pays the price.

7. Weaving it Together: The Act of Quiet Rebellion

My grandmother's kitchen wasn't just about food; it was about patience as an ingredient. When she soaked those lentils, she was teaching me that the best things in life cannot be rushed. As top wellness experts now recognise, our gut microbiome is like a garden. You cannot grow a garden with a blowtorch and a timer. You need water, time, and the right environment. By choosing slow cooking, soaking, and fermentation, you are giving your internal garden the chance to bloom. Slow cooking in a fast world is an act of quiet rebellion. It is a way of saying, "My health is worth more than a 10-minute convenience."

Awareness Note & Reflection

Take a look at your kitchen counter tonight. How many "instant" packets do you see? How many "10-minute hacks" have you fallen for this week?

Reflection Exercise:

1. Identify one "instant" food you rely on and see if there is a traditional, "slow" alternative you can try this weekend.
2. Observe how you feel after a "slow" meal versus an "instant" one. Is there a difference in your energy? Your mood?
3. Ask yourself: Am I saving time, or am I just rushing toward a health crisis?

Health is not cooked faster; it is built patiently, daily, and quietly.

The Stock Market of Weight Loss

Picture this: a humid afternoon in South Mumbai, where the salt-thick air of Marine Drive wraps around you like a heavy, wet blanket. The Arabian Sea is a restless grey, whispering ancient secrets to the jagged skyline of Nariman Point. I am perched at a corner table of a nostalgic Irani café, the scent of *bun maska* and *cutting chai* hanging in the air, sitting across from Abhishek.

Abhishek is a hedge fund wizard; eyes as sharp as a surgeon's scalpel, a man for whom millions of dollars are like loose change in a pocket. He is the master of the long game, a sage of the Sensex. But today, his silver fork hovers over a plate of limp, steamed broccoli like it's a ticking time bomb about to detonate. "Kiran," he hisses, his voice cracking like a sudden roll of thunder over the Gateway of India, "four kilos. I shed four kilos in two weeks of pure, unadulterated grit. Then, one sinful piece of *paneer tikka* at a client dinner last night; bam! I wake up, and the scale is 400 grams up. I'm already eyeing a 48-hour water fast to 'hedge' the storm. I feel like a pauper in my own skin, bankrupt of all my progress."

In that electric, humid moment, lightning strikes: Abhishek, the long-haul maestro of the markets, is treating his biological vessel like a wild, speculative penny stock. He has entered the Grey Zone; that foggy, psychological limbo between feast and famine, where the mist swallows logic and cravings clash like a fire alarm you can't shut off. He is chasing euphoric "green candles" of weight loss and dumping his progress in a panic at the first sign of a "red candle" on the scale. He is a sage investor in rupees, but a frantic, short-selling gambler in flesh and bone.

The Solar Surge of the Body's Economy

Welcome to the High-Voltage Circuit of Transformation. If your soul's barometer swings with every whisper of a bathroom scale, it is time for a radical audit. Your body is not a vending machine; it is a sophisticated, sun-drenched power grid, pulsing with energy cycles as radiant and intense as a summer noon.

1. The Volatility of the Flesh: In the high-stakes world of finance, volatility is the shared language of movement. Markets surge and slump like solar flares, inhaling hope and exhaling fear. Your weight odyssey mirrors this perfectly; its "Thermal Cycles" are often tragically mistaken for personal defeat.

- The Solar Flare (The Rapid Melt): You dive into a fierce, restrictive regimen. The initial flood of water weight exits the system. Triumph roars in your ears. You feel like a "Green Energy" Mogul, with praise shining down like golden sunlight from your colleagues. Your confidence hits a record high; you believe you've finally mastered the wild physics of biology. Warren Buffett? You're his desi heir, compounding "thinness" at record speeds. But much like a tech bubble, this initial surge is often driven by "Liquidity" (water) rather than "Solid Assets" (fat loss).

- The Brownout (Plateaus or Rebound): Then, the grid flickers. The scales freeze. Or worse, they spike after a single wedding feast. Shame surges like a power surge hitting a faulty fuse. Your habits begin to flicker; you skip your morning runs, you raid the hidden mithai drawer, and you find yourself lost in the darkness of self-doubt.

The echoes between the ticker tape and the waistline thunder clear:

- Panic Dump ↔ Crash Fast: When the market dips 2%, the amateur investor unloads everything in a frenzy. When your scale climbs 500g, you "panic dump" your nutrition, slashing your intake to a measly 800 calories. You are selling your long-term health to satisfy a short-term fear.

- FOMO Frenzy ↔ Trend Traps: Twitter hypes a new crypto moonshot, and you leap. Instagram flaunts the latest "Himalayan Ice Hack," and you snag the kit. The "Brownout" blurs your reason, making you forget that there are no shortcuts to a blue-chip body.
- Rally Chase ↔ Deficit Dash: You buy at the peaks, begging for just a bit more profit. You starve yourself deeper, chasing unsustainable 2kg weekly drops, blind to the fact that your muscle is melting away like ice under a desert sun. You are winning the trade but losing the portfolio.

2. The Silent Wreckers: Understanding Sentiment

Stock markets don't just move on complex data; they move on "sentiment." The collective mood of millions drives them. Similarly, our perceptions of our bodies shatter under the spell of the scale.

Top-tier wellness gurus preach "Mental Fitness" because they know your heart's ticker is synced to your weight's whims. When the "market" of your body crashes, anxiety claws at you. When you regain weight, the shame burns like a short-circuit.

Professional fund managers ignore their portfolios on an hourly basis because noise is not a trend. Yet, we interrogate our scales at dawn, letting a single number dictate whether we deserve to be happy.

The Hard Truth: Volatility is not the villain; your reaction to it is.

- Salt swells the tissues (The interest rate hike of biology).
- Stress simmers the hormones (The geopolitical tension).
- Sleep deprivation starves the metabolism (The liquidity crunch).

A 400g creep triggering a 48-hour thirst strike is not "discipline." It is the act of torching your life's vault over a single rupee's ripple.

3. The Power Grid Profiteers: Who Gains from Your Loss?

Just as brokerage platforms feast on the "churn" of frequent trades, the global weight-loss empire thrives on your cycles of failure. If everyone succeeded on their first attempt, the industry would go dark.

- 2025 Valuation: A staggering $18 billion to $165 billion.

- 2029–2033 Boom: Projected to reach a mind-bending $27 billion to $600 billion.

With a CAGR of 8–10%, this growth isn't driven by success; repeat flops drive it. Whether it is a $99 "detox" tea from a global brand or a ₹4,999 "miracle" ayurvedic kit from a local vendor, the result is a temporary water-loss "high." The moment you stop, the weight returns. You don't blame the product; you blame yourself. You head back to the bazaar for the "Upgraded Magic" version. They aren't peddling cures; they are peddling subscriptions to your own despair; charging you in every currency imaginable for a cycle that never ends.

4. The Global Map of Growth and Guilt

This bazaar spans the globe, but its stalls are etched differently in different locales.

- North America: Holds a 38% grip. They are the ultimate "churn queens," flipping through diets like fast fashion. They treat health like a quarterly earnings report; fast results or fire the CEO.
- Asia-Pacific: The fastest-growing flood of fitness anxiety. As traditional diets are replaced by processed "convenience," the panic rises.

- India's Pulse: Our market is expected to reach $7.93 billion in 2025. Our fitness realm alone is worth $257 billion. As our wallets get fatter, our mirrors feel frailer. We are trying to buy our way out of a problem we got ourselves into.

5. Speculator's Gamble vs. Investor's Anchor

To escape the cycle, you must ask: Are you a Speculator, or are you an Investor?

The Day-Trading Speculator (The Burnout)

- Hope's Haze: They look for "magic" ingredients over metabolic principles.
- Overkill: They have no "stop-loss" for their emotions. Every gram gained is a grave.
- The Quick Fix: Chasing a 5kg flash in a week, even if it means their thyroid is torched.

The Blue-Chip Investor (The Radiant Build)

- Patience: They understand that health compounding brews slowly, like the overnight fermentation of *idli* batter.
- Safeguards: They refuse to raid their "capital", their precious muscle mass.

- Steel Conviction: When the scales are stagnant, they stay rooted in their habits. They know that if the "fundamentals" (nutrition, movement, sleep) are strong, the "price" (weight) will eventually reflect the value.

A breakfast of Sprouted Moong Salad or Vegetable Poha isn't "disruptive." But these are the Blue-Chip assets that pay massive dividends in your silver years. Crash diets are "leverage lotteries"; you might see a 500% weekly "win," but the odds of a total health wipeout are nearly 100%.

Entering the Metabolic Recession

In the world of finance, a recession is a period of temporary economic decline during which trade and industrial activity are reduced. In the world of your body, a Metabolic Recession is far more dangerous because, unlike a central bank, you cannot simply print more "energy" once you have bankrupted your system. When you engage in "Panic Dumps" (crash dieting) or "Speculative Gambles" (extreme over-exercising without fuel), you aren't just losing weight; you are incurring High-Interest Metabolic Debt.

1. The Liquidation of Muscle (Asset Stripping)

When the body enters a severe calorie deficit, it looks for the most "expensive" assets to liquidate first. Muscle tissue is metabolically "costly"; it burns energy even while you sleep. To your body, muscle is like a high-maintenance luxury estate.

In a panic, your body performs Asset Stripping: it breaks down your muscle to save energy.

- The Investor's Loss: You might see the number on the scale drop (Short-term gain), but your "Basal Metabolic Rate" (BMR), your daily dividend of calories burned, tanks.
- The Result: You emerge from the diet smaller, but with a "broken engine" that requires even fewer calories to maintain, making future weight gain almost inevitable.

2. The Inflation of Hunger (The Hormonal Tax)

As you starve the system, your body's "Internal Revenue Service", the endocrine system, kicks in. It spikes Ghrelin (the hunger hormone) and slashes Leptin (the fullness hormone).

- This is Biological Inflation: the "cost" of feeling satisfied rises daily. Soon, a typical meal that used to satisfy you feels like nothing. You are now living in a state of permanent "Energy Poverty," where your brain is constantly screaming for a bailout of sugar and fats.

3. The Infrastructure Collapse (Bone and Immune Health)

Just as a nation might stop repairing bridges and roads during a depression to save cash, your body stops investing in "Non-Essential Infrastructure."

- Bone Density: Your skeleton becomes brittle.
- Immune Response: Your "Security Force" is defunded; you get sick more often.
- Hormonal Balance: For many, the reproductive system goes "offline" to save energy.

The "Compound Interest" of Recovery

Rebuilding a portfolio after a 50% market crash requires a 100% gain just to get back to zero. Rebuilding your metabolism follows the same brutal math. If you spend three months "Speculating" with a crash diet, it may take twelve months of "Patient Investing" (strength training and caloric maintenance) to repair the damage. You are essentially paying a 300% penalty for a few weeks of "looking thin" for a photo.

Investor's Insight: True wealth is not measured by how much cash you can burn in a week, but by the strength of your underlying assets. A healthy metabolism is a "Blue-Chip" asset that pays you back every single day of your life. Don't trade it for a "Penny Stock" miracle.

The Final Audit

Think about your money. You use spreadsheets and consult experts. You know financial losses are rebuildable. But health losses compound in the shadows. When you crash diet, you lose muscle and bone density. You are burning down your house to keep warm for one night.

The 15-Second Mirror

Close your eyes. Shut out the noise of the city. Recall your last desperate attempt to "hack" your body. Ask yourself:

"Would I stake my entire life's fortune on this fleeting flash, if I knew the ruin would stick forever?"

If you wouldn't take a "magic coin" for your life savings, stop reaching for the "magic pill" for your flesh. Cease the speculation. Invest in the core of your legacy. Your body is not a trade; it is the sun that powers your world. Treat it with the respect of a long-term investor, and the dividends will be a life lived in full light.

PART III: REDEFINING FITNESS

Fitness Is Not One Thing

"Your blood reports are perfect," my doctor friend said, tossing the folder onto the desk with a sigh that sounded like a tyre losing air. "Technically, you're a specimen of health. But looking at your face? Everything is wrong with your routine. You're fit on paper, but you're falling apart in person."

That line hit me like a cold shower at 4 a.m. It's the "Funny-but-Uncomfortable Truth" of our modern era. We live in a world where people can track their protein macros down to the last gram but haven't tracked their sleep hours in a decade. We see folks ordering a kale salad with the intensity of a monk, only to reward themselves with a triple-chocolate lava cake because "balance." We have thousands of people drinking cold-pressed green juice at 2 a.m. while scrolling through stress-inducing reels. We own resistance bands that have never actually resisted anything, except perhaps our desire to clean out the closet. After years of tried-and-tested methods, personal experiments, and coaching thousands, the realisation has finally landed: Fitness is not just the weight on the scale. Real fitness is a symphony of Emotional, Mental, and Physical health. If you are missing one, you aren't fit; you're just thin, or muscular, or "lucky" for now.

The Silent Puppeteers

We need to talk about the "Invisible Script" of our bodies. In our 20s, we are blissfully unaware of hormonal health. It feels irrelevant when you can survive on caffeine and pizza. But hormones don't shout; they whisper. They are the silent puppeteers of your metabolism. The effect of hormones is not very conspicuous at first, but it is severe by the time we learn what's happening. As we age, the definition of fitness changes. We realise that you cannot out-train a hormonal imbalance. When your Cortisol (the stress hormone) is chronically high, it acts like a biological bully, overriding your insulin and telling your body to hoard fat, specifically around the belly, as if a famine is coming.

Only if we had been so educated when we started! Most of us don't get the opportunity to go back in time to undo the actions whose consequences have now complicated our health. We spent our youth treating our bodies like a rental car, only to recognise in our 30s and 40s that we actually own the vehicle, and the parts are getting harder to replace.

Pillar 1: Emotional Fitness

I've seen people who can run marathons but can't sit through a five-minute conversation about their feelings without exploding. That isn't fitness. Emotional fitness is the ability to "lean in" to life.

Most of us walk around with a low-grade fever of resentment. We feel life is unfair. We find someone to blame: the boss, the ex, the government. But blame is a heavy backpack that slows your metabolic pace. Anger and resentment have never burned a single calorie of "bad energy"; they only increase oxidative stress. Many of us "run away" from life even while standing still. We experience things with a constant "Why me?" or "Why now?" background noise. But the fact that you are getting to experience life at all is the ultimate joy. I don't mean to trivialise your worries; I've had my share, but accepting your life, your fate, and your circumstances for what they are is the ultimate "workout" for your soul. When you stop resisting, you start living. Joy is a metabolic booster.

Pillar 2: Mental Fitness

Have you ever tried to eat a heavy meal while being chased by a lion? Probably not. But in the modern world, your "lion" is a deadline or a rude email. When you are stressed, your body enters "fight or flight." Blood flows away from your digestive tract and into your extremities so you can run or punch. If you eat in this state, your digestion and absorption suffer. Anything that improves your gut health has a positive impact on your mood. This is the Microbiome-Gut-Brain Axis.

The Sodium Propionate Secret

One of the most exciting research areas involves a metabolite called Sodium Propionate (NaP).

- What is it? It's a metabolite that aids digestion and helps produce Short-Chain Fatty Acids (SCFAs).
- The Brain Connection: It can cross the blood-brain barrier (the mesh of nerves that protects your brain) and regulate genes associated with mood and stress.
- The Clinical Edge: Studies show it can mitigate the physiological manifestations of depression, like altered colon length and weight loss.

You're already exposed to it in cheese and bread, but the real magic happens when you feed your gut the right fibres to produce these SCFAs naturally.

Food Options for a Fit Brain:

- Resistant Starches: Cooked and cooled potatoes or rice (the cooling creates the starch that feeds the good bugs).
- Fibrous Alliums: Leeks, onions, and garlic.
- The Polyphenol Punch: Dark berries and raw cacao.

Note: Depression is severe. Never experiment on your own; use this data to consult your medical expert.

Pillar 3: Genetics – The Blueprint vs. The Action

After we grapple with hormones, we admit the initiation of the problem often lies in our Genes. Your DNA is the deck of cards you were dealt, but your lifestyle is how you play the hand. We frequently blame "bad genetics" for a slow metabolism, but genetics are usually just "loaded guns"; it's your environment and habits that pull the trigger.

We had to have a whole lot of wins and failures to learn and unlearn this. We've admitted that the "One-Size-Fits-All" approach is a dangerous myth.

Pillar 4: Lifestyle

Let's address the elephant in the room: the Body Mass Index (BMI). I've written many times that this measure is wrong. It is a 19th-century metric for a 21st-century body.

I often think of physiques like Bruce Lee, extremely lean, muscular, and powerful. By BMI logic alone, even such a body could be misclassified as unhealthy. That is the limitation of BMI: it does not account for muscle mass. Body fat percentage and distribution are far more meaningful indicators.

- Visceral Fat: You get negative points for abdominal fat. This is the fat that wraps around your organs and pumps out inflammatory cytokines.
- Sleep: You cannot out-train a lack of sleep. Sleep is "cellular housekeeping." Without it, your brain screams for sugar because it lacks the energy to function.

Myth vs. Reality

Myth	**Reality**
One plan fits all: if it worked for your friend, it'll work for you.	Your microbiome and genetic expression are unique. A "perfect" diet for one is a "poison" for another.
Weight loss equals health.	You can lose weight through stress and illness. True health is about composition, energy, and mood.
Calories are the only thing that matters.	Hormonal response to those calories (Insulin, Cortisol) determines if they are burned or stored.

The Education We Need

Only if we understood all this before, that is the basic education we need. We must stop risking our bodies and our well-being for short-term results with hazardous consequences. We've had to unlearn the "shred" mentality to concede that fitness is a multi-dimensional puzzle.

Lean in; it is life. The opportunity to live it is worth the trouble. Many of us run from life with anger and resentment, but accepting and being joyful changes how we deal with everything. Anger never helped anyone heal. Don't let yourself get stressed by the challenges life brings. The opportunity to experience life itself is the ultimate joy. When you realise that your gut health influences your mood, your sleep influences your hunger, and your emotions influence your metabolism, you stop chasing a number and start chasing harmony.

15-Second Awareness Check

Stop. Close your eyes.

1. Scan your jaw: Is it clenched? (Release it).
2. Scan your breath: Is it shallow in your chest? (Take one deep, slow breath into your belly).
3. Scan your thought: Are you "running away" from this moment or "leaning in"?

You are now fitter than you were 15 seconds ago.

Muscle Matters More Than Weight

The air in the living room was thick with the scent of frying *puris* and the chime of laughter. It was my aunt's 60th birthday, and she looked, by all traditional standards, "perfect." She had maintained her wedding-day weight for three decades; a feat she wore like a badge of honour. She wore her vibrant silk saree with grace, moved nimbly between guests, and prided herself on eating only "clean, home-cooked meals."

Then, a glass of water was spilt.

It was a tiny puddle. A minor slip. In her 30s, she would have caught her balance. In her 40s, she might have bruised a knee. But at 60, despite her "ideal" weight, my aunt crumpled. The sound wasn't a thud; it was the sharp *crack* of a femur snapping like a dry twig. As we sat in the hospital, the doctor dropped a truth bomb that changed my perspective forever: "She's not overweight, but she's metabolically fragile. She has the skeleton of an 80-year-old because she has the muscle mass of a paper doll." This is the tragedy of the modern "healthy" woman. We have been conditioned to worship the scale, while our internal engines, our muscles, are quietly rusting away. We see our mothers and aunts managing household chores, wearing beautiful clothes, and eating home-made food, and we think they are "good." But beneath the surface, a dangerous shift in body composition is taking place.

A 19th-Century Relic

Let's start with a radical honesty session: The Body Mass Index (BMI) is a lie. Invented in the 1830s by a Belgian mathematician (not a doctor), BMI was never meant to measure individual health. It is a simple ratio of weight to height (Weight / Height^2). It is blind to the most important factor in human biology: Composition.

Imagine two men standing side-by-side. Both weigh 90kg. One is a sedentary office worker with a "soft" midsection; the other is a competitive athlete with thick, dense legs and a broad back. Their BMI will label them both as "Obese." This is the "Skinny-Fat" paradox. You can be thin on the outside and metabolically morbid on the inside.

Research Insight: Modern studies now show that Muscle Mass predicts longevity better than weight. In fact, some individuals classified as "obese" who possess high muscle mass actually outlive their "thin" peers who have low muscle density. Muscle is not just "meat"; it is a sophisticated organ that acts as a metabolic shock absorber.

Why Your Back Aches

I hear it constantly in social circles: *"Oh, it's just a little backache,"* or *"I'm just tired because I stood for 20 minutes cooking."* We have normalised physical frailty. We treat a sprained wrist or a slip in the bathroom as an "accident" rather than a symptom. But let's be clear: It is not normal to be exhausted after 20 minutes of standing. When you lack muscle, your skeletal system has no support. Your joints, ligaments, and spine take the full force of every movement. Think of muscle as the "suspension system" of a car. When the shocks are worn out, every tiny pebble on the road feels like a crater. For many women, their "suspension" has completely disintegrated, leaving their bones vulnerable to fractures from even the mildest falls.

The Biology of a Fall: In a body with healthy muscle, a slip triggers a rapid-fire neurological response. Muscles contract to stabilise the core. In a muscle-depleted body, that "signal" is slow, and the impact goes straight to the bone. This is why low muscle mass doubles your mortality risk. It's not the fall that kills; it's the inability of the body to protect itself during and after the impact.

The Body's Secret Pharmacy

Why does muscle matter so much for living to 100? Because muscle is our primary site for Glucose Disposal.

Every time you eat a bowl of rice or a piece of fruit, your blood sugar rises. In a muscular body, the muscles act like a giant sponge, soaking up that sugar to use as fuel. In a body with low muscle mass, that sugar has nowhere to go. It floats in the bloodstream, damaging arteries, or gets packed away as visceral fat around your organs.

Fun Fact

Well-researched data from top oncological wellness experts shows that high muscle density can cut cancer risk by approximately 30%. Muscle tissue secretes "myokines": small signalling proteins that have been shown to inhibit the growth of tumour cells and enhance the activity of "Natural Killer" (NK) cells in the immune system.

Redefining the Plate

The most common refrain I hear is: *"But I eat home-made food! Two vegs, dal, rice, chapati, dahi, and achar. The traditional thali!"*

While the traditional thali is culturally rich, we must be intellectually honest: it is often a Carbohydrate Bomb. Dal is a source of protein, yes, but it is roughly 70% carbohydrate. If your plate is 80% grains and lentils, you are fueling a body that isn't moving enough to burn it, and you aren't giving your muscles the building blocks they need to repair.

To change your composition, you must understand the Macros:

1. Protein (The Infrastructure): Without protein, your body cannot maintain muscle. As we age, we become "anabolic resistant," meaning we need *more* protein to get the same muscle-building effect.

2. Carbohydrates (The Energy): These should be earned. If you've been active, your muscles will welcome the glycogen. If you've been sedentary, that fat can accumulate.

3. Fats (The Hormone Spark): Essential for absorbing vitamins and keeping your brain sharp.

4. Fibre (The Gut Guardian): Crucial for clearing out the metabolic "trash."

The Protein Gold Standard

To gain or even maintain muscle, most top nutritionists now recommend roughly 1.2 to 1.6 grams of protein per kilogram of body weight. * For Men: Naturally more muscular due to testosterone, but often prone to "gut fat." They need consistent protein to maintain their metabolic lead.

For Women: This is critical. Estrogen helps maintain muscle; as it drops during menopause, muscle loss accelerates. You cannot "walk" your way out of this. You must "eat" and "lift" your way out.

The Workout Paradox

If I had a rupee for every person who said, *"I don't want to lift weights because I don't want to look bulky,"* I could retire today. Let's settle this: You will not accidentally become a bodybuilder. Building muscle is incredibly hard work. However, doing *only* cardio (like long walks) can sometimes be counterproductive. Excessive cardio without resistance training can lead the body to burn muscle for energy, making you a smaller, but flabbier, version of yourself.

The Prescription:

- Weight Training: 2–3 times a week. This "shocks" the bone into becoming denser and the muscle into becoming stronger.
- Cardio: For heart health and circulation, but it is the "accessory," not the "main event."

The Science People Don't Know

Deep in our genetics lies a protein called Myostatin, which acts as a brake on muscle growth. As we age, if we don't "signal" our bodies that we need our muscles, the brake stays on, and Sarcopenia (age-related muscle wasting) sets in. Recent research suggests that muscle isn't just about movement; it's about Cognitive Health. There is a direct link between grip strength (a proxy for overall muscle mass) and a lower risk of Alzheimer's. When you lift a weight, your muscles talk to your brain. If you stop moving, the conversation ends.

A New Vision for the "Lady of the House"

Think back to my aunt. If she had traded 20 minutes of her daily walk for 20 minutes of squats and lunges, her bone density would have been higher. If she had added a scoop of high-quality protein or increased her paneer/egg intake, her muscles would have been able to catch her when she slipped. We need to educate our families. It isn't enough to be "not fat." We need to be Strong. We need to move from the mindset of "staying a size" to "building a force Field."

Food Options for the Muscle-Minded:

- The Power Breakfast: Instead of just *poha* (pure carbs), try a moong dal chilla stuffed with paneer, or 3 egg whites and 1 whole egg.
- The Smart Lunch: Reduce the rice portion by half; double the dal and add a bowl of Greek yoghurt or grilled tofu.
- The Recovery Snack: A handful of almonds and a roasted chana mix, or a high-quality whey isolate if you are struggling to hit your protein targets.

Reflections

The next time you look in the mirror, I want you to look past the skin and the clothes. I want you to visualise the engine underneath. Is it robust? Is it capable? Or is it a fragile frame holding onto a number on a scale?

We must move away from the obsession with "weight loss" and move toward "muscle gain." Weight loss is often a subtraction of health; muscle gain is an addition of life.

My aunt is recovering now, but she's doing it the hard way, with physiotherapy and pain. You can choose to do it proactively. Change your composition. Balance your macros. Lift something heavy. Your future self, the one who wants to walk unassisted at 90, the one who wants to play with her great-grandchildren, the one who wants to live without the "normal" aches of ageing, is counting on you to start today.

The Muscle Score > The Scale

Your scale tells you your relationship with gravity. Your muscle mass tells you your relationship with time. Which one are you going to prioritise?

Acceptance Is the First Discipline

The mirror is often the most honest, yet most avoided, guest in our homes. We walk past it, suck in our stomachs, tilt our heads to a "favourable" angle, and spin a narrative. We tell ourselves that the fatigue is just "age," the breathlessness on the stairs is "just a heavy bag," and the tight waistband is "laundry shrinkage." We live in a beautifully decorated house of cards, praying that the wind never blows.

Recently, I was strolling through my neighbourhood when I noticed a newly opened bookstore. The smell of fresh ink drew me in. While browsing the children's section, I picked up a colourful board book about "Opposites." As I flipped through, I hit a spread that made me freeze. On one side, a cartoonish illustration of a "Fat" woman; on the other, a "Thin" woman.

In the world of a toddler, it was that simple. Black and white. Large and small. But as an adult, that page rang a bell so loud it vibrated in my chest. We have been socialised from the nursery to believe that "thin" is the destination and "fat" is the failure. We are taught to look at the silhouette, never the substance. This binary trap is exactly why so many of us live in denial. We chase the "thin" page of the children's book, even if that thinness is hollow and brittle.

The "Lucky" Survivor

I once knew a lady, Mishka, who lived by a philosophy of "minimalist survival." She was the neighbourhood enigma. She ate exactly one meal a day. Usually, it was a single paratha dripping with ghee or a quick sandwich. By some stroke of cosmic luck, she hadn't faced a major medical crisis yet.

But her "fitness" was an optical illusion. If you were to hug her, you wouldn't feel the bounce of muscle or the density of a nourished frame; you would feel the sharp, fragile outline of bones. Mishka flaunted her "thinness" with misplaced pride. She became a role model for the women in her circle. *"Look at me,"* she'd beam, *"I eat whatever I want once a day, and I'm fine!"*

But "fine" is a dangerous word. Mishka wasn't healthy; she was lucky. She was unknowingly playing a high-risk game with her health, relying on luck rather than building a strong physiological foundation. It's only by God's grace that she hasn't fallen or clipped a corner, because her body lacks the structural integrity to survive a stumble. Her story represents the biggest hurdle in the journey to wellness: the thick, impenetrable wall of denial.

The Anatomy of Denial vs. The Power of Acceptance

In my years of observing everyone from "old school" elders to my own peers, I've noticed a startling trend: rigidity is the enemy of longevity. Mention the word "Macros" (the balance of proteins, fats, and carbohydrates), and you'll often get a blank stare or a dismissive scoff. To many, it's modern gibberish; a "fad" for the young.

They believe that because they've "always done things this way," they are inherently right. They eat "well" by 1970s standards, ignoring that the soil, the stress levels, and the sedentary nature of 2026 are vastly different. They live in a state of "unconscious unfitness."

Acceptance is not giving up; it is waking up.

Giving up is a passive surrender: *"I'm old now, my knees are supposed to hurt."* Acceptance is an active realization: *"My body is currently unfit, my current methods are failing me, and I need help to change it."* Acceptance is the baseline. You cannot build a skyscraper on a swamp. Only when you admit, *"I have an unfit body, and I must work on it,"* does the real journey of education and balance begin.

Did You Know?

When the breath slows and the mind accepts reality, stress hormones reduce. This calm state naturally lowers emotional eating and cravings for quick, high-carb comfort foods. Acceptance doesn't just change the mind; it changes the body's chemistry.

Why Guilt is a Liability

We often see discipline as a burden, but for many women, the real burden is guilt. I remember a conversation with my cousin that perfectly illustrated this "martyr complex." She had been advised to drink fresh coconut water daily to remedy a severe deficiency.

Her response was heartbreakingly typical: *"I tried, but getting four coconuts every day for the whole family was getting too expensive, so I just stopped. I felt bad buying it just for myself."*

Her husband and children didn't have the deficiency. She did. Yet, she felt a crushing guilt taking that "luxury" for herself if she couldn't provide it for everyone. She prioritized the *feeling* of equality over her own health.

As women, we are socialized to be the last ones at the dinner table. But remember the flight safety briefing: Put on your own oxygen mask before helping others. If you collapse from exhaustion, who helps your kids? We must let our Intelligence Quotient (IQ) overtake our Emotional Quotient (EQ). Investing in your health, whether it's the cost of a coconut or the time for a walk, is not an "expense." It is an essential overhead for the business of living. If you survive, you can help them survive.

Stabilizing the Mind: The Nervous System as Your Foundation

Most people try to start a discipline with a chaotic mind. You cannot build a regime on a foundation of anxiety. You need a stable mind before you can practice discipline.

Our nervous system is like a biological musical instrument. If the strings are too tight, they snap. We need to "tune" ourselves into a state of calm focus before we can expect our bodies to follow a workout.

The Bhramari Breath

One of the most effective tools for achieving this is Bhramari Pranayama (The Humming Bee Breath). It is a direct line to your nervous system's "calm" setting.

1. The Seal: Close your ears with your thumbs and place your fingers gently over your eyes.

2. The Inhale: Take a deep, slow breath through your nose.

3. The Hum: As you exhale, keep your mouth closed and make a steady, low-pitched humming sound, like a bee.

4. The Sensation: Feel the vibration in your skull.

This vibration stimulates the Vagus Nerve, telling your brain, *"We are safe."* This transition from "Fight or Flight" to "Rest and Digest" is the secret to making discipline stick. By calming the nervous system, you stop the body from clinging to fat for "survival" and allow it to build strength.

Exercise is Not Leisure; It is a responsibility.

We need a radical reframing of "working out."

- Old View: Exercise is entertainment or something to do if there is "free time."

- New View: Exercise is a duty. It is a non-negotiable appointment with your future self.

You don't wait for "free time" to brush your teeth. You *make* time. Choosing a regime is about removing the guilt associated with self-care. When you exercise, you aren't "sneaking away" from your responsibilities; you are fulfilling the primary responsibility of maintaining the vehicle (your body) that carries out all your other duties.

The lifestyle change will ultimately benefit you and your family. You will be more active, stronger, and more independent. Your education in nutrition and macros becomes a helpful guide for your family, ensuring they don't have to rely on "luck" either.

From Luck to Logic

The lady in the bookstore's children's book was either "fat" or "thin," but life is lived in the muscles and the breath. The lady who eats one paratha a day and "flaunts" her thinness is a house of cards. Do not envy the "lucky"; emulate the disciplined.

Your fitness journey isn't a detour from your life; it is the fuel for it. Acceptance is the first discipline because it requires the most honesty. It is the moment you stop praying for health and start producing it.

A 15-Second Guided Pause

Before you turn the page, let's practice the first step of discipline.

- Inhale for 4 seconds. (Accept your current state)
- Hold for 2 seconds. (Commit to the change)
- Exhale slowly for 6 seconds. (Release the denial)

Accept this moment. You are here. You are starting. The next step is education; understanding what your body truly needs; and creating a daily, non-negotiable responsibility hour for movement.

Food, Mood & Focus

Have you ever noticed how a high-stakes board meeting suddenly feels less like a battlefield and more like a brainstorming session once the platter of grilled appetisers arrives? Or why, after a screaming match with a relative, do you find yourself sprinting to the smallest room in the house, the toilet?

It’s not just "nerves," and no, your cousin isn't just making an excuse to skip the dishes. It’s the Gut-Brain Axis in full, rowdy action. This is the unseen telecommunications network where your breakfast talks to your brain, and your boss's passive-aggressive email talks directly to your bowels.

As someone raised in a vibrant North Indian family, I've seen it all. In our house, we don't do "subtle." We have loud, operatic reactions to everything, from a burnt paratha to a wedding announcement. For years, I watched family members rush to the bathroom during heated arguments or anxious situations. I'll admit, I used to roll my eyes. I believed they did so to run away from the situation or that they were making an excuse.

I couldn't have been more wrong. Recently, I dove deep into the science of the Enteric Nervous System (ENS), often called our "second brain." I realised that the gut is essentially a giant tuning fork for our emotions. Our mind doesn't just "influence" our gut; it dictates its rhythm. When we are mentally or emotionally compromised, even the cleanest, most organic kale salad can feel like a stone in our stomach. You can be as careful as you want with your food, but if your mind is in a state of civil war, the state of your mind will impact the effects of that food on your body.

The Chemistry of the Kitchen Table

Food is far more than calories; it is a psychological lever. Think about it: why are the biggest business transactions in the world closed over lavish dinners rather than in sterile cubicles? Because the right food softens the edges of a hard bargain. The mood in a family can be literally lit up with food. A tense conversation about finances or grades can be transformed into a positive, enjoyable exchange if the palate is satisfied.

The Golden Rule of Digestion: Food consumed in a happy mood is metabolised with precision. A "sulking body," however, shuts down its digestive fires. When you eat while stressed, your body enters "Fight or Flight" mode. Your brain yells, *"Forget the biryani! There's a tiger in the room!"* and shunts blood away from your digestive tract and into your legs so you can run.

Research Flash: Did you know that about **90–95% of our serotonin** (the "feel-good" hormone) is produced in the gut? If your gut is unhappy, your brain literally lacks the chemistry required to be "happy." It's hard to be a Zen master when your colon is staging a protest.

The Forgotten Nutrient

Before we talk about what goes in your mouth, we have to talk about what goes in your eyes. We often forget that Light is Food.

In the modern world, we are "malnourished" when it comes to natural light. We spend our lives under the flicker of LED bulbs, wondering why we feel sluggish.

Setting	Lux (Light Intensity)	Impact on Mood/Focus
Indoor Office/Home	**200–300 lux**	**Drowsiness, low serotonin**
Outdoor Daylight	**10,000+ lux**	**High focus, resets circadian rhythm**

The 15-Second Exercise: Stop right now and ask yourself: *"Where did your eyes meet light today, the screen or the sky?"*

Your morning sunlight isn't just for a tan; it's a biological "reset button" for your circadian rhythm. Stepping outside for just 10 minutes signals your brain to stop producing melatonin and start producing cortisol and serotonin. It's the ultimate, free "Focus Supplement." Download a Lux Meter App today; it's a fantastic awareness tool to see just how "dark" your indoor life really is compared to the sky.

The Secret Weapon

If you are chasing good health, it is hard to throw a rock and not hit the topic of gut health. But among the sea of probiotics, there is one unsung hero: Butyrate.

So what is butyrate, and how does it affect you?

Butyrate is a short-chain fatty acid (SCFA) that your gut bacteria make when you eat the right kind of food. It is produced in your colon when friendly bacteria ferment dietary fibre. Think of it as premium fuel for your gut cells, known as colonocytes. These cells line your intestinal wall, forming a barrier that keeps harmful substances out of your bloodstream.

When butyrate is present, your gut barrier stays strong, reducing inflammation. When levels drop, the barrier weakens, leading to what we often call a "leaky gut." But there is more. Butyrate helps regulate inflammation and improves insulin sensitivity. It even influences your brain through the gut-brain axis. It is known to increase Brain-Derived Neurotrophic Factor (BDNF), a molecule that enhances learning, mood, and memory. In simple words, a healthy gut helps build a healthy brain.

Decision Fatigue

By the time the sun begins to set, most of us have already spent our mental "currency" for the day. From the moment you wake up, you are bombarded with a relentless stream of choices: which email to prioritise, how to phrase a sensitive text, what route to take to work, or how to handle a sudden deadline. We make hundreds of these micro-decisions before noon, and each one acts like a small leak in a bucket. By 6:00 PM, that bucket is empty. This isn't a lack of willpower; it is simply "Decision Fatigue." When your brain is exhausted from a day of navigating complexity, it loses its ability to filter. This is why the person who ate a disciplined salad at lunch finds themselves mindlessly reaching for a bag of chips or scrolling through a screen for hours in the evening. You aren't being lazy; your brain has run out of the fuel required to say "no."

The Cost of Saying 'Yes' Too Often

The weight of our evenings is often determined by the "yeses" we hand out during the day. We accept promotions without considering the lost sleep they entail, we take on extra office responsibilities to seem capable, and we succumb to family expectations and social obligations to avoid conflict. This "emotional tax" accumulates quietly, but health is always the one that pays the bill. When you over-commit, you trade your internal peace for external approval. By the time you get home, the sheer volume of "yeses" you've served to others leaves you with nothing left for yourself. This exhaustion pushes you toward sugar for a quick energy boost, toward screens for a numbing escape, and toward a heavy silence because you no longer have the words to engage. "I'll start tomorrow" isn't a sign of weakness; it is a survival mechanism for a mind that has been stretched too thin by the world's demands.

The Corporate "Food Pivot": A Real-Life Lesson

A few years ago, we hit a massive crisis at work. The atmosphere was thick with gloom and finger-pointing. I decided to change the traditional "serious" reaction to a courageous one by ordering high-quality, "guilt-free" food from the best place in town.

The shift was instantaneous. The motivated employees handled the situation positively because they weren't battling a sugar crash from oily snacks. During my own exams, I always preferred guilt-free meals to increase concentration. Fitness is a mental game, and we have to master the tricks of the trade to play it well.

To maximise butyrate and keep your mood stable, follow these **Three Pillars**:

1. **Eat More Fibre:** Your gut bacteria need raw material. Focus on onion, garlic, asparagus, broccoli, and leafy greens.

2. **Add Resistant Starch:** When you eat **cooked and cooled rice or potatoes** (or green bananas), you are consuming resistant starch. Your gut bacteria love it and increase butyrate production naturally.

3. **Include Fermented Foods:** Yoghurt, kefir, kimchi, and sauerkraut, which add the beneficial bacteria needed to maintain a microbiome capable of producing these mood-boosting SCFAs.

4. **Healthy Fats:** Butter from grass-fed cows naturally contains small amounts of butyrate. Enjoy it!

The "No-Go" Zone: Avoid processed foods, sugar, refined carbohydrates, and additives. They are the "party poopers" of your microbiome.

No Two Guts are the Same

Each body is unique. One person's stress leads to a constipated body, while another's leads to loose motions. The same body will react to similar situations in several ways based on the current situation each time. It's a dynamic process, and we can't give up. We have to be strong mentally and emotionally, but we must also understand our bodies.

The Symphony of the Sky and the Stomach

We started with the image of family members rushing to the toilet during an argument. We now realise they weren't making excuses; their gut was simply echoing the mental stress.

Fitness isn't just about the size of your waist; it's about the resilience of your spirit. By combining **natural light** (the sky/sun), **fibrous/fermented foods** (the gut), and **emotional awareness** (the mind), you become the conductor of your own biological symphony.

Next time you face a challenge, whether it's a university exam or a business merger, remember the "Focus Signals." Look to the sky for light, look to your plate for fibre and fermented goodness, and remember that a happy gut is the foundation of a courageous life.

Master the tricks of the trade. Look up from your screen, feed your microbes, and play the mental game well.

Fitness for Self, Not Approval

Imagine, for a moment, the heavy, humid air of a city zoo. The usual background chatter and rustling popcorn bags suddenly snap into a chilling silence, followed by a collective gasp. A man has fallen into the tiger enclosure. The massive Bengal tiger, a five-hundred-pound engine of pure muscle and predatory instinct, begins to stalk toward him. The man is small, terrified, and instinctively huddling into a ball; the universal posture of "prey."

But here is a fact that sounds like a tall tale, yet is rooted in the deep psychology of wildlife behaviour: experts say that the animal would not have been able to drag the man away if he had simply found a way to stand tall. If he had climbed onto a nearby bench or a sturdy table, making himself appear physically taller than the beast, the tiger would have hesitated. In the wild, height is an evolutionary signal of authority and danger. The sight of a man standing tall would have scared the tiger into retreat. It seems absolutely unbelievable, but the psychological "height" of the man could have tamed the beast's instinct.

In the year 2026, we find ourselves in a different kind of enclosure. We aren't facing a feline, but we are facing a

Monster Culture; a relentless, prowling beast of digital influencers, algorithmic manipulation, and a desperate hunger for external validation. To survive this modern zoo, we have to stop huddling in fear. We have to stand still and stand tall in front of this monster culture to survive.

The AI Flood: When Your Phone Becomes a Puppet Master

We live in an age of unprecedented access. Information is everywhere, flowing like a broken fire hydrant, but much of it is "tainted" water. There is so much Internet access, so many views, and so many influencers that you truly never know what is right and what is wrong. Here is the technical reality of how you are being hunted: the more you search for information, whether it's "flat stomach in five days" or "miracle supplements", the more the AI-generated social media links will flood toward you. The algorithm is a mirror; it reflects your insecurities back at you. If you get fooled by every advertisement or flashy video coming your way, you will quickly become a physical and mental wreck. This industry doesn't just want your money; it wants your agency. The format of the fitness-influencer world works on specific chemical reactions in our brains. By triggering dopamine through the promise of a "miracle" and then playing on our fear of being "not enough," they can make us puppets. They effectively handicap our minds, leaving us unable to draw a line between a healthy habit and a dangerous obsession. It is a very dangerous situation where the data being collected on you is so humongous that platforms can use it to get you to give them whatever they want.

The "Miracle" Hustle: High Costs and Broken Promises

The modern influencer has replaced the qualified professional with "quick fixes" that are, in reality, dangerous traps. These individuals position themselves as "Doctors," "Advisors," or "Elite Coaches," guaranteeing results that defy the laws of physiology. They sell you herbal oils, mystery supplements, or registration fees for "exclusive" clubs. Because we are humans, and because our health is so deeply tied to our self-esteem, we are emotionally vulnerable. We are tempted to pay huge sums of money because we are looking for a lifeline. I have seen the damage this causes:

- The High Stakes Loss: A close friend of mine was duped into losing 50,000/- over such a "hack." The coach promised a complete transformation but delivered nothing but a generic PDF.

- The Detox Trap: Another acquaintance lost 12,000/- in the name of a "detox diet" that resulted in nothing but severe dehydration and fatigue.

The bitter pill to swallow? These commitments are not documented. They are not legally bound. When the "miracle" fails to manifest, you have no recourse. You are fooled and duped at the same time, and the emotional fallout is often worse than the financial one. Our behaviour becomes so irrational during these phases that even a well-wisher, a spouse, a sibling, or a long-term family doctor looks like an enemy to us because they are trying to burst our "hope" bubble.

The "Like" Trap: Validation from the Unknown

Another trap, perhaps more subtle but equally lethal to our peace of mind, is the quest for Likes from unknown people on social media. Think about the absurdity of this: an approval from an unknown, long-lost person on social media can impact you, positively or negatively. It can literally make or break your day. We have outsourced our happiness to the "thumb" of a stranger.

When we train or eat for the "Gram," we aren't building health; we are building a brand. This makes us incredibly vulnerable.

We are playing a game where the rules are set by an algorithm that wants us to stay insecure, because insecure people keep scrolling, and scrolling people keep buying.

Reclaiming the "Bench": Internal Authority

To survive the "Tiger" of modern culture, we need to be sensible and take back control of our lives. This control must include both Body and Mind. We have to work on ourselves for our personal benefit, not to show anyone else.

1. Educate Yourself (The Real Power): The only way to stop being a puppet is to understand how the strings work. Educate yourself on the basics of biology and nutrition. When you know how insulin actually works, an advertisement for "belly-melting herbal oil" doesn't look like a miracle; it looks like a comedy.

2. Seek Real Sources: If you need heart surgery, you don't go to an influencer with a nice smile; you go to a surgeon. Why should your daily health be any different? Take advice from a real source, such as a qualified doctor or a nutritionist. Real expertise is often boring and involves "consistency" and "balance," which is exactly why it doesn't always go viral.

3. Internal vs. External Validation: If your workout only happens when you post a selfie, who are you really working for? You must shift your focus inward. The "Like" those matters is the feeling of your heart beating strongly, your lungs taking in deep breaths, and your joints moving without pain.

The "Taller Man" Strategy: Standing Still

The "Monster Culture" thrives on your movement; your clicking, your searching, your frantic switching from one fad to another. To scare the tiger, you must stand still.

Standing still means:

- Drawing a Line: Deciding that your health is not for sale to the highest bidder on your feed.
- Logical Auditing: Asking, "Is this person a qualified doctor, or do they just have great lighting?"
- Protecting Your Well-wishers: Realising that the people who have known you for twenty years probably have your best interests at heart more than a "coach" who has known you for twenty seconds.

The Self-Respect Menu (Food for Focus)

When you are training for yourself and not for approval, your food choices change. You stop looking for "skinny teas" and start looking for sustenance.

- The Satiety Secret: Instead of a "detox juice" (which is often just sugar water), choose fibre-rich whole grains like steel-cut oats or millets. They keep your blood sugar steady so you aren't making irrational, impulsive decisions online.
- Brain Fats: Nourish your "internal authority" with walnuts, flaxseeds, and fatty fish. These provide the DHA your brain needs to maintain focus and resist the "handicapping" effects of social media.
- The Power of Probiotics: A healthy gut produces the neurotransmitters that keep you emotionally stable. A bowl of homemade curd (*dahi*) is worth more for your mood than a thousand digital likes.

The Posture of Power

We return to the man in the enclosure. He is no longer huddling. He is standing on the table, looking the tiger in the eye, asserting his presence. The Internet is a humongous ocean of data, and if you are not careful, you will drown in it. But if you stand tall on the foundation of education, internal authority, and qualified advice, the monster of "approval culture" loses its power. You become the master of your own chemistry, not a puppet on a digital string. Work on yourself because you deserve to feel good. Work on yourself so you can live a long, vibrant life. Work on yourself because your body is the only home you will ever truly own. Everything else, the likes, the trends, the herbal miracles, is just noise.

Reflection Question

Put your phone face down, close your eyes, and ask yourself this:

"If I were the last person on Earth and no one was watching, how would I move my body today? Am I building a temple for my soul, or a stage for a stranger's approval?"

PART IV: EXPERIENCE, STRESS & REAL LIFE

Everything I Tried

The year was 2004. I stood in front of my bedroom mirror, holding my breath hard enough to see stars, trying to zip up a pair of "slim-fit" jeans that were clearly designed for a mannequin. Like many teenagers, I wanted to walk onto my college campus with confidence, the kind that turns heads and makes you feel seen. That desire quietly became a mission: not just to be like someone, but to be someone everyone noticed.

This is the strange dilemma of adolescence: the tug-of-war between attraction and validation. We begin chasing an external idea of perfection: sharper features, leaner bodies, and proportions dictated by trends rather than biology. Instead of nourishing our bodies for the lives we want to live, we often treat them as problems to be fixed.

And so began my long relationship with diets.

The Great Indian Diet Cycle

If persistence alone guaranteed success, I would have mastered health decades ago. I tried almost everything; each new method promising transformation, discipline, and control.

Keto came first. It demanded complete devotion while banning carbohydrates entirely. For months, my meals revolved around fats and proteins while I stared longingly at rotis and rice. The results came quickly and disappeared just as fast. The moment carbohydrates returned, so did the weight. Keto, while effective in the short term, proved unsustainable for an Indian lifestyle rooted in dal, grains, and balance.

Then came OMAD (One Meal a Day); extreme fasting packaged as discipline. Twenty-three hours of restraint, one hour of consumption. Social life vanished, irritability took over, and hunger dictated mood. What I later learned was critical: prolonged fasting spikes cortisol, the body's stress hormone, signalling scarcity. When the body believes it is under threat, it holds onto fat. What looks like control is often physiological resistance.

Next were detoxes and liquid diets; green juices, liver cleanses, and celebrity-endorsed shakes. The promise was purification; the reality was dehydration. The liver does not need “cleansing teas.” It is already a sophisticated detoxification system. Most cleanses simply flush water, electrolytes, and energy, leaving fatigue behind.

Across all these attempts, the pattern was consistent: initial success, rapid rebound. Every “quick fix” worked briefly and failed permanently.

The Illusion of the Perfect Body

The idea of the “ideal body” changes faster than fashion trends. One decade glorifies extreme thinness; another celebrates curves and strength. Chasing these shifting standards is exhausting and futile. Much of what we admire on screens and social media is curated, filtered, and staged. Lighting, angles, and editing create bodies that don’t exist in real life. This realisation was freeing. The problem was not my discipline or effort. The problem was the benchmark.

Health had been replaced by appearance.

From Diets to Systems

Years of trial led to one clear conclusion: there are no permanent shortcuts. Sustainable health requires systems, not extremes.

Over time, I arrived at three foundational pillars that actually work.

1. Movement as a Trinity: No single form of exercise is sufficient on its own.

- Yoga builds mobility, balance, and mental calm.
- Weight training increases muscle mass, the body's metabolic engine. More muscle means higher calorie burn even at rest.
- Cardio or dance strengthens the heart and improves endurance.

Together, they create resilience, not just weight loss.

2. Macro Awareness: Instead of counting every calorie, understanding macronutrients changed everything.

- Protein: 1.2–1.5 grams per kg of body weight supports muscle and recovery.
- Fats: Essential for hormonal balance and skin health.
- Carbohydrates: The brain's primary fuel, especially when chosen wisely (oats, brown rice, whole grains).

Food stopped being the enemy and became fuel.

3. Redefining Fitness Benchmarks: The scale is a poor judge of health. Real indicators are functional:

- Can you carry groceries without strain?
- Can you climb stairs without breathlessness?
- Do you wake up without chronic aches?

A pain-free, energetic body is the real achievement.

A Moment of Clarity

At a destination wedding, after weeks on a restrictive "quick fix" diet, I was thin, but depleted. Low energy, hair fall, irritability. Nearby, a woman in her sixties danced for hours, ate mindfully, and radiated vitality. She wasn't chasing numbers; she was enjoying life.

That moment reframed everything.

The goal was not to look smaller; it was to live better.

What the Science Confirms

Once I moved beyond trends and into research, the conclusions were consistent:

- Muscle memory is real. If you've trained before, your body regains strength faster.
- The gut-brain connection matters. Nearly 90% of serotonin is produced in the gut. Chronic under-eating affects mental health.
- NEAT (Non-Exercise Activity Thermogenesis); daily movement like walking, standing, fidgeting; often burns more calories overall than a single gym session.

Health is cumulative, not episodic.

The Wisdom We Ignore

During a low-calorie phase, an older aunt once looked at my tiny salad and said, *"Itna kam khaoge toh ghar kaise chalega?"* At the time, I dismissed it. Years later, I understood: energy is capacity. Without it, nothing functions: career, relationships, or joy.

You cannot be a show-stopper without stamina.

No Finish Line Exists

Fitness is not a three-month project or a cinematic transformation arc. There is no "wrap." The body keeps adapting every day. What works is simple, not easy: Patience. Consistency. Discipline.

Sleep matters. Recovery matters. Repetition matters.

Don't chase a finish line that doesn't exist. Build habits that last. Choose energy over exhaustion. In the long run, people won't ask what diet you're on; they'll ask why you look so alive.

In the story of your life, don't let fads write the script. You are the director. Choose longevity over illusion.

When Life Gets in the Way

"You would be lucky if your body were your only concern."

Let that sentence sit with you. Scroll through Instagram, and it appears that people have only three responsibilities: sipping matcha in aesthetic cafés, performing flawless headstands, and sleeping nine uninterrupted hours on luxury sheets. Health looks effortless there. But you and I live in the real world. In reality, your body is only one tenant in a crowded apartment complex called life. It is an important tenant; it pays the rent of existence, but it is not alone. There are other loud residents: family, career, finances, ageing parents, household responsibilities, and constant uncertainty. When life applies pressure, it rarely does so gently.

Sometimes life doesn't knock. It breaks the lock. And when that happens, the green smoothie is always the first casualty. This chapter is not about perfect workouts. It is about what happens when deadlines collide with domestic responsibility, when emotional load and mental stress create a chemical storm that no amount of treadmill time can erase.

The 6:15 AM War Room

Let's look honestly at a typical day in the life of the modern Indian woman. It does not begin with a gratitude journal. It begins with an alarm.

The day starts at 5:30 AM. You wake before sunrise, not as a mother alone but as a logistics manager. School-going children need to be ready. The bus arrives at 6:45 AM, which means the entire kitchen operation must run with military precision. Two snack boxes per child must be packed before 6:15 AM. Teenagers are bottomless pits with legs, and underfeeding them turns them into emotional zombies. Breakfast is prepared, lunchboxes are packed, water bottles filled, uniforms checked, and instructions issued.

Then comes the commute. You are not listening to music. You are coordinating remotely with the nanny.

"Did the milkman deliver?"

"Lunch for the kids is sorted?"

"Tuition at 4 PM, don't forget."

"I've soaked the dal; tell the cook to make dinner."

By the time you reach work, you have already run a marathon. That tight chest and shallow breathing are not imagination. They are biological signals.

The Invisible Villain

As you sit in traffic, worrying about work, school, finances, and family, your body is flooded with cortisol.

Cortisol is not the enemy. Historically, it was our survival hormone. When a predator appeared, cortisol released glucose into the bloodstream, enabling fight or flight. The response saved lives. Today, the predator is different. It is your boss, the traffic jam, your child's academic pressure, and the fear of financial instability. The problem is that you cannot run or fight these threats. The glucose released has nowhere to go.

Here is the critical truth behind stress-related weight gain: When cortisol remains chronically high, the body enters famine mode. First, fat storage increases, specifically visceral fat around the abdomen. This location is strategic, close to the liver, allowing quick energy conversion if danger persists. Even clean food will be stored when stress remains unresolved. Second, cravings intensify. Cortisol suppresses leptin, the satiety hormone, and increases ghrelin, the hunger hormone. After stress, the brain seeks dopamine. This is why cravings lean toward sugar and salt, not vegetables. Third, sleep collapses. You fall into bed exhausted but wake at 3 AM. The nervous system is stuck in survival mode, leaving you tired but wired.

The Golden Handcuffs

Let me tell you about my neighbour, Ritusha.

She was intelligent, ambitious, and placed in a senior role at a top finance firm. At the same time, she was raising teenage children who needed emotional presence more than material comfort. She was offered a promotion with a 60% salary increase. It required six working days and constant travel. On paper, it was ideal. In reality, she was already dealing with acidity, hair fall, insomnia, and stubborn weight gain. She sat across from me, exhausted, asking if she should take it. I told her not to.

The money would remain in the bank while her health deteriorated. A 60% raise is meaningless if it results in a 100% rise in cortisol. Working relentlessly while managing adolescent children is not building a future; it is dismantling the present.

The Turmoil of Unidentified Goals

Why do we do this? Often, we are chasing goals we never consciously chose. Titles, salaries, possessions; scripts written by society. Chronic stress removes clarity. Everything feels urgent. Emails, laundry, meetings, and messages all demand equal attention.

When everything is urgent, nothing is important.

The Reset Button

The solution is not greater effort. It is conscious disconnection.

Introspection: Not coffee breaks, but honest evaluation. Ask whether the pace is sustainable. If earnings are consumed by medical bills and exhaustion, the balance sheet is already negative.

Meditation: Not spirituality, but nervous system regulation. Meditation lowers cortisol and restores clarity. It teaches the brain that not every stimulus requires a reaction.

Nutrition for stress: Under stress, digestion weakens. Raw salads worsen bloating. Instead, rely on foods that calm the system.

Cashews provide tryptophan and magnesium, supporting serotonin production. Gond katira cools internal heat and reduces acidity. Curd rice with hing and jeera supports the gut-brain axis and calms anxiety. A teaspoon of ghee at night lubricates digestion and improves sleep.

Everything Will Fall in Place

Prioritising health does not always mean waking at 4 AM to exercise. Sometimes it means sleeping longer. Sometimes it means declining a promotion. Sometimes it means choosing a peaceful body over a swollen bank balance. When you choose balance, the fog lifts. Cortisol drops. The body feels safe, and weight begins to normalise naturally.

Life will always interfere. That is inevitable. But you are the driver. You can slow down, change direction, or stop. Just don't let the engine burn out before the journey is complete.

Control the Mind, and Cravings Follow

The clock strikes 4:00 PM. You are sitting at your desk, and suddenly, it's there; the "phantom" smell of hot, buttery samosas or that specific brand of hazelnut chocolate. You aren't hungry; you had a nutritious lunch two hours ago. But your mind has just staged a coup. It's no longer your brain; it's a high-definition billboard for junk food. We've been sold a lie: that every "craving" is a "wish," and that a life well-lived is one where every wish is granted. We think, *"If I don't eat this, I'm depriving myself of happiness."* But let's get naturalistic; since when did a deep-fried dough ball become the gatekeeper of your joy?

The "Wish" Delusion: Ego vs. Reality

We often enter a silent, exhausting Ego Tussle with ourselves. Influenced by a "treat yourself" culture, we start to believe that our "wishes" (read: cravings) are sacred. We tell ourselves that we are "achievers" and "bosses" who deserve to have whatever we want. But here's the twist: when you give in to a craving that harms your body, you aren't being an "achiever." You're being hijacked. You are sacrificing your long-term health for a 15-second tongue party. We treat our cravings as if we're living in a Pixar movie where we can eat five cupcakes and still have the waistline of a Disney princess.

Newsflash: Your body isn't an animation. It’s a biological machine that keeps the score. True ego-strength isn't about having the "power" to buy the cake; it’s about having the clarity to recognise you don't actually want it.

Cravings: The Body’s Telegram

Cravings are not a sign of a "weak" character; they are signals. Think of them as encrypted telegrams from your cells, helping your audience feel seen and understood in their body's messages.

- The Chocolate Telegram: Usually means your body is screaming for Magnesium.
- The Salty Chip Telegram: Your body is likely dehydrated or missing Electrolytes.
- The "Eat Everything" Telegram: Your Cortisol (stress hormone) is through the roof.

When your macros are balanced, with enough protein, healthy fats, and complex carbs, and your mineral levels are topped up, these "telegrams" stop arriving. A well-nourished body is a quiet body.

The Bermuda Triangle of Cravings

Cravings love a messy mind. If your brain is a cluttered closet of deadlines, family drama, and Instagram-induced FOMO, your "Mindfulness" gets buried under the junk. When you are sleep-deprived, your brain's 'CEO' (the Prefrontal Cortex) goes on vacation, leaving the 'Toddler' (the Amygdala) in charge of the snacks. Incorporate mindfulness practices like deep breathing or brief meditation during stressful moments to help slice craving intensity by 30–50%. Why? Because it brings the CEO back to the office, empowering you to manage cravings consciously.

The 15-Second Circuit Breaker

Before you rip open that packet, run this diagnostic check. It takes 15 seconds and saves you 500 empty calories. Ask:

1. H: Hunger: Is my stomach physically empty, or is my mouth just bored?
2. T: Tiredness: Do I need a cookie, or do I actually need a 20-minute nap?

3. S: Stress: Am I eating this to "numb" a feeling?
4. B: Boredom: Am I just looking for a hit of dopamine because this Zoom call is dull?

The Story of the "Happiness" Muffin

I once worked with a high-performing professional, Rahul. Rahul was convinced that his 5:00 PM blueberry muffin was the "highlight of his day." He told me, *"It's my one wish, I can't give it up."*

I asked him to do one thing: Eat the muffin mindfully. No phone, no emails, just him and the muffin. Focus on each bite- notice the texture, flavour, and aroma. Chew slowly and savour the experience. This simple practice helps you distinguish between true hunger and craving, making it easier to break the cycle of mindless eating. On Day 3, Rahul called me. *"It's weird,"* he said. *"I acknowledged the muffin tastes like cardboard and fake sugar. I only liked the smell of the bakery because it reminded me of leaving work."*

The "wish" was a fake. Once he decluttered his mind and separated the feeling (relief of finishing work) from the food (the muffin), the craving vanished. He wasn't losing happiness; he was gaining freedom.

The Smart Swap Sheet

If you are struggling to tell the difference between a biological need and a mental "want," use this guide to outsmart your brain:

The "Harmful Want"	The Real "Biological Need"	The Smart "Body-Love" Swap
Fizzy Sodas	Calcium / Hydration	Sparkling water with a squeeze of fresh lime
White Bread / Pizza	Nitrogen / Energy	A bowl of roasted Makhana (fox nuts) or Paneer
Sugary Candy	Phosphorus / Chromium	A handful of berries or a piece of local fruit

Late Night Cereal	Sleep / Tryptophan	A cup of warm turmeric milk (Haldi Doodh)

Declutter for Clarity

Cravings are like uninvited guests at a party. If your house (your mind) is messy and loud, they'll stay and wreck the place. But if your house is calm, organised, and well-lit, they concede they don't belong and leave on their own, inspiring your audience to feel hopeful about their ability to cultivate a peaceful mind. Eating mindfully isn't a chore; it's a superpower. It's the actualisation that you don't need to "control" your cravings with a whip and a chair; you just need to observe them. When you balance your body with the right minerals and your mind with the right focus, you admit that the most "achiever" thing you can do is to feed your body only what makes it legendary.

Stop wishing in a dreamworld. Start living in your best body.

Drugs, Devices & the 2026 Fitness Wave

Imagine walking into a high-school reunion or a wedding in early 2025. You scan the room and notice something striking: people who struggled with their weight for decades are suddenly svelte. Your former colleague looks like a marathon runner. Even the local baker seems to have shrunk. This isn't just a sudden burst of collective willpower; it is the **GLP-1 revolution** in full swing. By the end of 2024, the world had already spent a staggering **$30 billion** on these medications. By now, in 2026, they are as common as a morning multivitamin. But as we celebrate this "metabolic shortcut," we must look closer. Are we building lasting health, or are we just renting thinness?

The Silent Revolution: How It Works

You've likely never heard of **Joel F. Habener**. While he recently passed away, his seminal work created the foundation for the drugs we now know as Ozempic, Wegovy, or Mounjaro. These aren't just "diet pills"; they are sophisticated hormone mimics.

GLP-1 (Glucagon-like peptide-1) is a hormone your gut naturally releases to tell your brain, *"Stop! We are full."* In 2026, we've mastered the art of amplifying that signal. When you take these peptides, several critical things happen within your biology:

- **The Brain Signal:** It communicates profound satiety. Suddenly, the "food noise", that constant mental chatter about what to eat next, that magnetic pull toward the pantry at 10 PM, is muted.
- **The Insulin Anchor:** It raises the amount of insulin your body makes after eating, helping manage blood sugar effectively and ensuring your cells utilise energy rather than storing it as fat.
- **The Sugar Shield:** It lowers the amount of sugar released into your blood, creating a more stable internal environment.
- **The Slow-Mo Stomach:** It slows the rate at which food passes through your stomach. This prevents sharp blood sugar spikes and keeps you feeling fuller for much longer.

The 2026 fitness wave isn't just about vanity or fitting into a smaller pair of jeans. Rigorous scientific research has shown these drugs offer benefits that go deep beneath the skin, affecting the very core of our longevity:

- **Heart Health:** Clinical trials have demonstrated a significant reduction in cardiovascular risks, lowering the incidence of heart attacks and strokes.
- **Better Rest:** We are seeing massive improvements in **obstructive sleep apnea**. As visceral fat (the dangerous fat around your organs) decreases, airways clear, and thousands are finally waking up feeling truly refreshed.
- **Metabolic Reset:** For those with chronic lifestyle issues, these drugs offer a "floor" to stop a downward health spiral, providing the breathing room needed to implement long-term changes.

The Reality Check

One of my close friends recently took a GLP-1 drug. The transformation was rapid; the weight seemed to melt away. But as the months passed, she looked tired rather than fit. Her skin lost its glow, and her energy levels plummeted. Why? Because the medication was doing all the heavy lifting of appetite regulation, but she had **no durable habits** to buffer the inevitable rebound.

This is the danger of the 2026 wave. The medication manages the hunger, but it doesn’t lift weights for you. If you haven't changed your behaviour by the time you stop the drug, the body will regain the lost fat almost instantly. You end up back at square one, often with a worse body composition than before. To avoid this, you must fight the "Muscle Tax":

1. **Low Protein Intake:** Because the drug makes you feel full so quickly, many people stop eating enough protein. Without these essential building blocks, your body begins to scavenge its own muscle tissue for amino acids.

2. **No Resistance Training:** If you don't engage in strength training, your body has no "reason" to maintain its muscle mass. In a calorie deficit, it will burn muscle for fuel just as readily as fat, leading to a "skinny-fat" appearance and a crashed metabolism.

3. **Irregular Sleep:** Weight loss is a metabolic renovation. Without 7–8 hours of quality sleep, your body stays in a state of stress, making it harder to maintain progress and easier to regain weight once the pharmaceutical assistance ends.

Myth vs. Reality

In the 2026 landscape of metabolic health, it is vital to separate fact from fiction regarding the new wave of weight-loss medications. While many believe these drugs are a "fix-all" solution, the reality is that they only manage hunger; true health remains a product of lifestyle. Simply reducing the portion size of poor-quality food isn't enough; your body still requires high-quality nutrients to maintain bone density and the health of your hair and skin. Furthermore, far from being the "easy way out," using these medications actually demands *greater* discipline to perform the resistance training necessary to prevent muscle wasting. Ultimately, without a foundation of durable habit change, the weight is likely to return the moment the injections stop, proving that pharmaceutical assistance is a bridge, not a permanent destination.

The 2026 Toolkit

We are no longer guessing in the dark. The 2026 wave is defined by high-tech integration. **AI-driven apps** now act as 24/7 health coaches, predicting when your blood sugar might dip based on your sleep patterns and stress levels. **Wearables** have moved beyond simple step counting; they now track "Muscle Quality" and "Metabolic Flexibility" in real time.

Furthermore, we are seeing a beautiful integration of **mental health** into weight loss. For the first time, we are widely acknowledging that "Food Noise" is often "Emotional Noise." Modern clinics now pair prescriptions with behavioural therapy, recognising that to change the body permanently, we must first address the internal triggers that lead to overeating.

A word of serious caution: With the massive popularity of these drugs in 2026, the market is currently flooded with "grey-market" frauds and counterfeit peptides. Always be extremely cautious about your source. Never jump into trying new medical interventions without proper clinical guidance and a prescription from a licensed professional. Your health is not something to be outsourced to an unverified online vendor.

There are too many conflicting goals in modern life: socialising, travel, high-pressure work, and constant stress.

For those who are genuinely unable to build a consistent life habit due to underlying biological or metabolic hurdles, this medicine can be a lifesaver. It provides a biological "reset." However, you must realise that you are essentially replacing a lifetime of good habits with a lifetime of medication.

For those who want to embark on the journey to build true, lasting health from the ground up: **Failing is fine.** Do not be afraid of the struggle. Learn from the times you could not achieve your goals. Disaggregate why it happened. Was it the environment? The stress? The lack of preparation?

Break your journey down to the smallest, simplest tasks that you can do without friction. Eat one less bite of processed food. Walk ten more steps today than you did yesterday. Pick up a slightly heavier weight. Slowly build your capacity.

Discipline and consistency are infectious. They don't just affect the number on the scale; they shape your character and who you are as a person. The real miracle of 2026 isn't found in a needle or a high-tech wearable; it's in the discipline you cultivate in your daily life. Whether you use medication as a bridge or choose the path of pure habit, the ultimate question remains: **Who do you want to become?**

Choosing Awareness Over Perfection

Imagine it is 7:00 PM on a Tuesday. You are standing in front of an open refrigerator, staring at a half-wilted bunch of coriander and a lonely carton of yoghurt. Your brain feels like a smartphone with forty apps running in the background. Then, that heavy, dreaded question hits: *"What should I cook tonight?"* If you've ever felt a surge of irritation or sheer exhaustion at that moment, you aren't alone. When we talk to any woman, especially in the context of Indian joint families, they all say the same thing: Deciding what to cook takes more time and effort than the actual cooking. It sounds like a casual complaint, but it is a sensitive, high-stakes decision. You have to balance what everyone likes, what is healthy, which ingredients are actually in the pantry, and how much time you have left before the kids lose their minds. This daily "mental load" affects the moods and energy of the entire house. When we don't have a plan, we give in to hunger pangs and cravings, landing us in a nutritional blunder.

This chapter is your permission slip to stop trying to be perfect. Most people don't fail at health because they lack knowledge or motivation; they fail because they are decision-fatigued.

1. Batch Cooking vs. Decision Fatigue: The "Auntie" Method: We often think "meal prep" means spending Sunday afternoon packing 21 identical plastic containers with steamed broccoli. It's not. Batch cooking is actually about reducing the number of times your brain has to sweat. I remember one of my aunts who lived in a bustling joint family. She had a legendary pre-decided timetable taped to her fridge. It was her constitution. If it was Monday, Lunch was *Mutter Aloo*, and Dinner was *Dal Rice*. This exact timetable continued for decades. Whether it was on purpose to avoid lengthy, circular discussions with her daughter-in-law or simply tradition, it worked. For ten years, Mondays were "sorted." Right or wrong, no one bothered to argue because the decision was already made.

When you plan and decide in advance, the clutter in your head vanishes. Once the "what" is settled, the "how" is easy. You can disconnect from the kitchen stress and focus your precious mental energy on other important work.

The Library of Treasure: I have another friend who treated her kitchen like a world-class archive. She had a "Library of Recipes", a massive collection of box files. One for Soups, one for Chicken, one for Biryanis. There were 50 files! When it was time to eat, she didn't "think"; she just chose an item, and her house help referred to the notes. We can do the same! By creating a library of recipes where the Macros (Proteins, Fats, Carbs) and Calories are already calculated, we choose based on our daily requirements. No math, no stress, just execution.

2. Removing Decisions, Not Food Groups: In the world of "fad diets," the first thing people do is demonise a food group. "No Carbs!" "No Sugar!" "No Fats!"

But restrictive rules are like a tight spring; the harder you pull, the more violently they trigger a "rebellion" inside you. This section reframes the problem: The enemy isn't the potato; it's the decision overload. Awareness beats restriction every time. Instead of following rigid, fragile rules that make you feel guilty for eating a piece of fruit, you should design "Default Choices." The Concept: A default choice is a pre-set path. If you are at a restaurant, your "default" might be a grilled protein and a side of greens.

The Result: You aren't "dieting"; you are simply following a system you built for yourself. This leads to consistency without the heavy baggage of guilt.

3. Sustainable Consistency Over Short-Term Perfection: Health is often sold to us as a light switch: it's either On (perfect execution) or Off (total collapse). But perfection is fragile. A late meeting, a flat tyre, or a sick child can "flip the switch" to off, leading to the "Screw it, I already ruined the day" spiral. Please reframe health as a dimmer switch (The Dial). A "10" on the dial is a perfect workout and a balanced, home-cooked meal.

- A "3" is a 10-minute walk and a simple bowl of lentils.
- The Secret: A "3" is infinitely better than a "0."

Progress does not require intensity; it needs attention. Small, repeatable actions, like choosing water over soda or batch-cooking one protein compound over time. Perfection is a sprint that leaves you breathless; consistency is a walk that takes you across the country.

4. The "Emergency Backup" Protocol: Even with the best "Auntie-style" timetable, life happens. You need an Emergency Meal. This is a decision-free safety net that requires zero prep and zero thought.

- Examples: A specific protein shake, a rotisserie chicken from the store, or a pre-portioned frozen healthy meal.
- Why it works: It prevents the desperate "I'll eat anything I get my hands on" moment. When you are exhausted, your

willpower is drained. The Emergency Protocol saves you from making a choice you'll regret tomorrow.

5. Emotional Awareness vs. Hunger Awareness: To choose awareness, you must know what you are feeling. There is a considerable difference between Physical Hunger (your stomach needing fuel) and Stress Hunger (your brain seeking a dopamine hit to cope with a bad day). Try the "10-Minute Pause." Before acting on an impulsive craving, set a timer for 10 minutes. Observe the feeling. Ask: *"Am I hungry, or am I just bored/angry/tired?"* You aren't trying to stop the craving; you are just noticing it. This simple act of awareness takes the "remote control" out of your impulses' hands.

6. The 5-Hour Rule: Educating Yourself: We cannot depend on others' advice all the time. To be truly free, we must educate ourselves on the basics of nutrition.

- The Habit: Read or learn about nutrition for one hour a day. That's 5 hours a week of building your "Awareness Muscle."
- The Goal: When you understand the rights and wrongs of healthy eating, you can proceed with confidence. You become an expert on your own body.

You don’t need perfection; you need awareness. Instead of judging yourself for “low willpower,” you’ll recognise decision fatigue for what it is. You’ll see how simple, repeatable meals create freedom, not boredom, and why systems work better than struggle. Most importantly, you’ll learn to course-correct without guilt, building habits that quietly support you for decades.

PART V: INTEGRATION & PEACE

The Environment Within and Around You

Why Calm Minds and Safe Circles Change the Body

Imagine a race where ten frogs are tasked with climbing a steep, slippery wall. As they start, the crowd begins to jeer: "It's too high! You'll never make it! Look at your legs; they aren't strong enough!" One by one, discouraged by the noise, the frogs lose heart and tumble down except for one. This little frog keeps climbing, steady and unfazed, until he reaches the very top. The secret? He was deaf. He couldn't hear the demotivation. He didn't have to "overcome" the negativity because he never let it into his internal environment in the first place.

In the world of fitness, we are often that frog, but with one major disadvantage: we can hear everything. We hear the harsh criticism in our own heads and the "harmless" jokes from friends. We try to climb the wall of health while carrying the weight of shame. This chapter is about learning when to plug your ears, how to change the channel in your head, and why the people you share your lunch with might be more important than the calories on your plate.

1. The Body: Your Only Lifelong Roommate: We spend so much time trying to "escape" our bodies through dieting or distraction, but here is a grounding truth: **No one can separate us from our bodies.** Partners, friends, and even jobs can come and go, but your body is the only person who will be with you from your first breath to your last. Often, we have a laundry list of expectations. We want a different nose, flatter abs, or thinner legs. But as the saying goes, "You cannot heal a body you hate." Approving of your body isn't about being "perfect"; it's about a shift in attitude. If you identify the positives, perhaps your legs are strong enough to walk you to work, or your arms allow you to hug your children; you create a foundation of cooperation. When you work on your weaknesses from a place of acceptance rather than disgust, the body stops resisting and starts responding.

2. The Biology of "Not Enough": Why does self-criticism sabotage your workouts? It's not just "mental"; it's biological. Constant "cribbing" (complaining) and negative self-talk attract the wrong energy and keep your nervous system in survival mode. When you look in the mirror and think, "I look terrible," your brain perceives a threat. It releases cortisol, the stress hormone. High cortisol levels are like a "Do Not Disturb" sign for fat loss; they disrupt sleep, slow down

digestion, and trigger intense cravings for quick energy (sugar).

The Survival Loop:

- **Step 1:** Shame/Self-Criticism → **Step 2:** Stress Response → **Step 3:** Poor Sleep/Fatigue → **Step 4:** Emotional Eating → **Step 5:** More Shame.

Fitness is 100% emotional and mental. If the mind isn't calm, the body won't feel safe enough to change.

3. Gratitude: The Ultimate Performance Enhancer: Most people think gratitude is just "being nice." In reality, it's a strategic tool. There are two primary motivational techniques: **Appreciation** and **Shame**.

- **Appreciation** is like fuel. It sustains.
- **Shame** is like a whip. It might make you run today, but it leaves scars and leads to burnout.

Research shows that gratitude practices improve consistency more than willpower ever could. When you are thankful for what you have, you lower internal resistance. You aren't "forcing" yourself to the gym; you are taking your body out for movement because you value it.

I Recently Figured Out…

"I used to think I needed to be stricter to see results. It turns out, I was more disciplined on the days I felt thankful, not the days I felt guilty."

4. The Contagion of Habits: "Show Me Your Friends...": There is a famous proverb: "Show me your friends, and I will show you your future." In the world of wellness, this is scientifically backed. Humans are biologically wired to mirror the behaviour of those around them. This is known as **Social Contagion**.

If you hang out with four people who prioritise protein, movement, and early sleep, you will likely become the fifth. If you hang out with people who constantly complain, eat mindlessly, and mock health efforts, you will struggle to stay on track, no matter how much "willpower" you have.

5. Dealing with the "Crabs in a Bucket": We all know them; the people who call you "self-obsessed," "over-conscious," or "boring" because you chose a salad or went for a morning run. **Here is a secret from the future:** The very people criticising your discipline today are the ones who will come to you in ten years and say, "I wish I hadn't given up. I wish I had continued as you did." Their mockery isn't about your "obsession"; it's

about their own insecurity. When you change, it holds up a mirror to their lack of action. Like the frogs at the bottom of the wall, they want you to come back down so they don't feel left behind. Be the deaf frog. Stay focused on the goal.

6. Why Groups Win (The Power of the Circle): Why do group-based programs or family-wide health shifts work so much better than solo efforts?

1. **Reduced Friction:** You don’t have to argue about where to eat if everyone values health.

2. **Subconscious Influence:** Habits are contagious. If your "tribe" prioritises health, you do it to fit in, which is the strongest human urge.

3. **The Safety Net:** When you have a bad day, a supportive circle pulls you up; a toxic circle gives you a shovel to dig deeper.

Feature	Toxic Environment	Supportive Environment
Reaction to Progress	Mockery/Sarcasm	Encouragement/Curiosity
Talk Topics	Weight/Flaws/Others	Energy/Strength/Growth
Effect on Stress	High (Defense Mode)	Low (Safety Mode)

7. Real-Life Snapshot: The Tale of Two Routines: Consider two people: Ananya and Rahul. Both eat 1,800 calories and walk 10,000 steps.

- **Ananya** lives in a home where her parents mock her "health phase", and she spends her nights scrolling through Instagram influencers, feeling "less than."

- **Rahul** has a group of friends who hike on weekends and a partner who cooks healthy meals with him. He starts his day by acknowledging one thing his body did well.

The Result? Rahul sustains his routine for years with 20% effort. Ananya burns out in three months because she is fighting a war on two fronts: her inner critic and her outer circle.

Mini Practices (Very Low Effort)

1) 15-second Gratitude Scan: Before getting out of bed, name one thing your body did for you without being asked.

2) The Circle Check: Notice your WhatsApp groups or frequent callers. Ask yourself: Who makes healthy living feel lighter, and who makes it heavier?

3) The "Deaf Frog" Technique: When someone mocks your discipline, don't engage. Stay focused and keep moving forward.

Integrated Insight: Care grows faster in appreciation than in criticism. Being hard on yourself may feel productive, but it rarely leads to lasting results. Treat your body as a lifelong partner. Build on your strengths, work gently on your weaknesses, and choose your company wisely. Often, the habit that needs changing isn't food or exercise; it's your inner dialogue and the voices you allow around you.

Learning Over Following: What Fitness Finally Means

Have you ever had one of those mornings where you wake up, and for a split second, everything feels perfect? The house is quiet, the sunlight is hitting the floor just right, and you feel… light. You aren't thinking about your to-do list, you aren't worrying about the calories in your breakfast, and you aren't scolding yourself for skipping the gym yesterday. For that one beautiful moment, you are just **happy**. You are at peace. Then, reality kicks in. You remember the "rules." You remember that some fitness guru on the internet said you should be drinking lemon water at 5:00 AM, then running 3 miles, then drinking a kale smoothie that looks like it came out of a lawnmower. Suddenly, that feeling of peace vanishes, replaced by a familiar, heavy weight in your chest. The "fight" begins again.

I spent most of my life in that fight. I thought that to be fit, I had to be slightly miserable. I felt that "happiness" was something I would earn *after* I reached a certain weight or mastered a specific pose. I was always waiting for the finish line so I could finally relax and be at peace.

But here is the secret that changed my entire life: **Happiness isn't the reward for being fit. Happiness is the fuel that gets you there.**

We talk a lot about "Zen mode," and sometimes that sounds like you need to go live on a mountain and eat nothing but air. But fundamental Zen mode is actually much funnier and simpler than that. It's the feeling of eating a piece of chocolate and actually *enjoying* it, rather than doing math in your head about how long you'll have to run to "burn it off." It's the peace of mind that comes when you acknowledge your body isn't a problem to be solved, but a friend to be looked after. When you finally stop fighting yourself, something phenomenal happens. Your shoulders drop. Your breath gets deeper. You start to smile more, not because you've reached some "perfect" goal, but because you've finally stopped following a map that was making you lose.

I want this final part of our journey together to feel like the best kind of conversation. Imagine we are sitting on a porch, the sun is setting, and the pressure of the world has just… evaporated. We aren't here to talk about "discipline" or "willpower"; those words are too loud and too tired. We are here to talk about **freedom**.

We are moving into a space where fitness means feeling good in your skin right now, not ten pounds from now. We are moving into a space where your mind is calm because you finally trust yourself more than you trust a celebrity's meal plan.

This is the part where you get to take off the heavy backpack of "shoulds" and "musts" that you've been carrying for years. We are going to find that sweet spot where health and happiness aren't just roommates, but best friends.

So, take a sip of whatever you're drinking, let out a big sigh, and let's get into it. This isn't just about "learning" anymore. This is about finally coming home to yourself.

The Morning of 2026: A Vision of Becoming

I want you to take a deep breath and look at the calendar for a moment. We are a few weeks into 2026. For many of us, this date used to feel like a distant science-fiction movie, but here we are. I was sitting in my kitchen the other day, staring at a little note I'd tucked into my planner. It had two words on it: Hiraya Manawari. It's a beautiful, ancient phrase that translates to: "May your dreams come true," or more deeply, "May what you envision become real." As I look around at the messages being shared this year, I see the same prayer in everyone's eyes. We are all whispering it: "Please, let my family stay healthy. Let us be free from financial stress. Let this be the year of 'forever happiness.'" We all want that "better, successful life." But if I've learned anything from years of struggle, it's this: You cannot pray your way into a healthy body while following a map designed for someone else.

The Illusion: My Life as a Professional "Follower"

Let's be honest. I spent most of my life trying to achieve the impossible without actually knowing the facts. I was running after an illusion. I call it the "Filtered Mirage." You know the one; the body that looks perfect under ring lights, the energy that never seems to dip, and the diet that consists only of colourful berries and expensive powders.

I have learned the hard way that when you chase an illusion, you eventually trip over your own feet. There wasn't a diet fad in the entire industry that I didn't get tempted by. If there was a "magic" cabbage soup that promised to melt five kilos in five days, I would be in the kitchen chopping cabbage until my fingers were sore. If there were a rule saying I should only eat between 4:00 AM and noon while standing on one leg, I probably would have tried it. Every single time a new "guru" appeared with a shiny new promise, I told myself: "This is it. This is the one. This is where my life finally starts." And every single time, I failed. I'd start with such intensity on Monday, feeling like a warrior, and by Thursday night, I was sitting on my kitchen floor, crying over a bag of chips, feeling like a total disaster. I thought the problem was my willpower. I thought I was "broken."

But I really have to thank the universe that I was lucky enough to understand, well in time, that the problem wasn't me. The problem was that I was a "follower." I was waiting for someone else to give me the answers to my own body. I finally realised that real fitness is happiness. The more I lead a happy and disease-free life, the more fit I actually am. Fitness doesn't have an end line. It's not a trophy you win and then put on a shelf. It's a journey. It is what accountants call a "going concern"; it's something that never stops moving.

Why "Copy-Paste" Fitness Always Breaks

We live in a world where we are taught to copy others. If your neighbour buys a new car, you want to know the brand. If your friend loses weight, you want the name of her trainer. But your body is not a car, and it's not a set of blueprints.

The Problem with One-Size-Fits-All

Why do those 30-day "shred" plans or influencer diets almost always fail? Because they ignore you.

Imagine trying to wear someone else's prescription glasses. For them, the world is crystal clear. For you, everything is a blurry mess, and you end up with a headache. That's exactly what happens when we copy someone else's routine.

The Mismatch: You might be trying a high-intensity workout you saw on Instagram, but you're a parent who hasn't slept more than four hours a night for three weeks. Your body doesn't need "intensity"; it needs "recovery." By pushing yourself because a "plan" told you to, you aren't getting fit; you're getting exhausted.

The Vanishing Act: Following is external. Learning is internal. If you follow a plan, you're just a passenger. If the driver (the trainer or the diet) disappears, you're lost. If you learn why your body reacts to certain foods, you become the driver.

Dulling Your Own Voice: Blindly following a set of rules makes you deaf to your own body. You stop asking, "Am I actually hungry?" and start asking, "Does my paper say I can eat now?" You stop noticing that your knees hurt or that you feel cranky after a certain meal because you're too busy trying to be a "good student" of a bad system.

The Burnout Cycle: Success from imitation is always short-lived. You can force yourself to follow a strict rule for three weeks, but the moment life gets "real", when you have a deadline, a sick family member, or just a bad day, the rule breaks. And when the rule breaks, we blame ourselves.

Did You Know? A massive 95% of people who lose weight on a strict diet regain it all back. It's not because they are lazy. It's because they followed a "result" instead of learning a "principle." The following tells you what to do. Learning tells you why it works, and what to do when things go wrong.

I Recently Figured Out…

"I stopped asking 'what should I eat?' and started asking 'what suits me?' The moment I stopped looking at other people's plates and started looking at how I felt after a meal, everything changed. I wasn't fighting anymore; I was just living."

Why the Industry Wants You Confused

Let’s have a little "real talk" about the fitness world. I’m not here to point fingers at specific trainers or brands, but we need to see the industry for what it is.

The fitness industry is a giant business. And like any business, it loves repeat customers. Here is the secret: Dependence is profitable. Independence is free.

The Profit in Confusion

If you are confused, you are a customer. If I tell you that one week "fat is the enemy" and the next week "carbs are the poison," you stay in a state of panic. And when you are in a panic, you buy things. You buy the "fat-burning" tea, the "carb-blocking" pill, or the new "detox" kit.

If you actually learned the basic facts, that local, seasonal food is your best friend and that a 20-minute walk is better than a 2-hour gym session you hate, you wouldn't need to buy a new "secret" every month.

The Rule-Changer Game

Have you noticed how the "rules" of health seem to change every Tuesday? One day, eggs are a superfood; the next day, they are a heart attack in a shell. This constant shifting keeps you chasing the next answer. It keeps you a "follower."

It's important to realise that this isn't about blaming anyone. It's just how the system is built. But you don't have to play that game anymore. You can step out of the waiting room.

Learning makes you independent. Following keeps you dependent. When you depend on others for your happiness or your health, you are giving away your power. We have to take responsibility today for what we are and what we want to be. Blaming the "latest fad" or the "bad trainer" won't make us fit. Taking charge of our own learning will.

The 15-Second "Why" Test

Next time you are about to start a new health "trend," stop for fifteen seconds. Ask yourself:

"Do I know why I am doing this, or am I just doing it because someone with a nice smile told me to?"

Don't judge yourself. Just notice the answer. If the answer is "I don't know why," then it's time to stop following and start learning.

What Fitness Actually Means

If you've read this far, you might be thinking, "Okay, if it's not the six-pack or the cabbage soup, what is it?"

We need to reframe fitness. It's not a goal you reach; it's a relationship you have with yourself. It is a "going concern." You can never come to a point of "perfect health" and say, "Okay, I'm done, I can eat whatever and stop moving." In fact, as we get older, our journey becomes even more rigorous, but it feels easier because we have more awareness and knowledge.

The Four Pillars of Real Fitness

Let's look at what being "fit" actually looks like in real life:

1. A Body That Doesn't Break Easily: Real fitness is about being "sturdy." It means if you catch a common cold, your body fights it off. If you have a long day, your back doesn't ache. It's about a disease-resistant body, not a fragile one that only looks good in photos.

2. A Body That Supports You: Your body should be your best friend, not your enemy. Fitness means your body says "Yes" when your life says "Go." Yes to carrying your groceries, yes

to playing with your kids, and yes to dancing at a wedding without needing to sit down after every song.

3. A Calm Mind: True fitness is having a mind that is regulated and calm. If you are constantly stressing about every calorie or feeling guilty about a piece of cake, you aren't "fit"; you're in a state of mental exhaustion. Fitness is when your mind and body are on the same team.

4. A Lifestyle That Lasts: If you can't see yourself doing it when you're 70, it's not fitness. It's just a phase. Real fitness is the way you live your life every single day, not just for the three weeks before a beach vacation.

The Ultimate Fact: Fitness is seasonal and personal. What works for you in your 20s will change in your 40s. What works when you are on holiday will not work when you are at a high-pressure job. And that is perfectly normal.

Putting It All Together

We've talked about many things in this book, but as we conclude, I want you to see that these weren't separate ideas. They were all pieces of the same puzzle.

1. Muscle is more critical than weight: Stop fighting the scale. Your muscles keep you moving and support a healthy metabolism.

2. Awareness is more important than control: Control is about force and "willpower," which constantly runs out. Awareness is about listening to your body, which lasts forever.

3. Calm is more critical than discipline: We are told fitness is a "war" or a "fight." But when your attitude changes, it stops being a fight and finally starts working.

4. Consistency is more important than intensity: Doing a little bit every day beats doing a "perfect" workout once a month.

These aren't just tips; they are the facts of a happy life. When we stop running after the "impossible" and start doing what is right for our mind and body, the results come naturally.

Fitness in the Real World

Fitness isn't something that happens in a gym. It occurs in the grocery store, your kitchen, your office desk, and your bed. A fit life doesn't look the same every year, and it shouldn't.

How Fitness Adapts to You

1. During the Busy Work Years: Fitness might mean taking the stairs, drinking enough water, and learning how to say "no" to late-night stress-eating. It’s about keeping your energy steady so you don’t crash at 3:00 PM.

2. During the Parenting Years: Fitness is about functional strength. It’s about being able to lift a sleeping toddler without hurting your back. It’s about finding 10 minutes of "me time" to breathe so you can be a calmer parent.

3. During Travel or Crisis: Fitness is about adaptability. It’s about knowing how to make the best choice at a gas station or a hotel buffet because you understand your body's needs.

As we age, fitness becomes about independence. It’s about keeping our bones strong and our balance steady so we can keep doing the things we love for as long as possible.

Myth vs. Reality

Myth: Fitness has an end goal (like "I'll be fit when I lose 10 kilos").

Reality: Fitness is a lifelong relationship. It’s a journey that adapts to your life, not the other way around.

Fun Fact: Did you know that people who define fitness as "feeling energetic" or "sleeping better" actually stay active for many more years than people who only focus on "looking thin"? When the goal is happiness, we don't want to quit!

The Final Shift: From Prisoner to Architect

As we close the cover on this journey, please take a long, deep look at the person you were when you started Chapter One.

For years, you were told that fitness was a tax you had to pay for existing. You were told it was a "war" you had to win, a "grind" you had to survive, and a "body" you had to borrow from someone else's social media feed. You spent so much time fighting your cravings and apologising to your reflection that you forgot one simple, breathtaking fact: **Your body is the only home you will ever truly own.**

The struggle was exhausting because you were trying to build a house using someone else's blueprint. But today, the fight ends. Not because you've reached a finish line, but because you've recognised there is no finish line—there is only the beautiful, ongoing process of living well.

Your New Sovereignty

From this moment on, you are no longer a "follower" waiting for permission to feel good. You have become the architect. When you stop obsessing over the "how much" and start understanding the "why," the heavy chains of the fitness industry simply fall away.

- **You are the expert:** No guru, no app, and no influencer knows the rhythm of your heart or the hunger of your cells better than you do.
- **Silence the noise:** You don't need a louder coach; you need a quieter mind. When you listen to your body instead of the headlines, the "impossible" suddenly becomes common sense.
- **Freedom is the goal:** Real fitness isn't being able to fit into an old pair of jeans; it's being able to wake up without a heavy heart and a list of self-criticisms.

The 15-Second Transformation

I want you to do something radical. Forget every number, every calorie, and every "should" that has ever haunted you. Strip it all back until it's just you and your breath.

Now, finish this sentence in your mind: **"From this day forward, my health belongs to me because _______________."**

Is it because you want to dance at your daughter's wedding? Is it because you deserve to feel energetic at 4 PM? Or is it simply because you are tired of being unhappy? Whatever your reason is, it is more powerful than any diet plan ever written.

The Horizon is Yours

When fitness stops being a fight, it finally starts working. It stops being a chore and starts being your secret weapon. It becomes the energy that fuels your career, the patience that heals your relationships, and the peace that lets you sleep soundly at night.

You aren't "restarting" on Monday. You aren't "trying again." You are simply living—with awareness, with facts, and with a heart that finally knows it is enough.

The door is open. The air is fresh. The power is yours.

Go live.

A Final Heart-to-Heart: From My Kitchen to Yours

Thank you, truly, for trusting me with your time and your journey. Over these chapters, we've walked a long path together, and I want you to know that this book was never meant to be a cold manual or a list of "dos and don'ts." It was written as a conversation between two friends, sitting across a table, both just trying to figure out how to live our best, most vibrant lives.

I've been where you are. I've felt the frustration of the "Monday reset," the confusion of the latest diet trends, and the exhaustion of trying to live up to someone else's definition of "perfect." But the biggest lesson I can leave you with is this: **You don't need a guru, because the only real expert on *you* is sitting in your chair right now.**

I hope you walk away from these pages feeling lighter, not just in body, but in spirit. I hope you've realised that you have the power to stop the fight and start the flow.

As you move ahead in 2026 and beyond, keep asking "why." Keep leaning into your curiosity. Keep growing into the person you've always envisioned being. But most importantly, please, **keep being happy.** Don't let a calorie count or a missed workout steal your joy. Protect your peace, cherish your health, and remember that a happy heart is the actual engine of a fit body.

That is where real fitness lives. That is where your new life begins.

Before you close this chapter, pause for a moment and notice the voice you speak to yourself with. You talk to yourself about more than to anyone else in your life. What does that voice do? Does it replay your last mistake, the failed project, the missed deadline, the sharp word you regret, the promise you broke to yourself, and then punish you for it?

For most of us, that voice is not compassion but correction. Not patience, but pressure.

Yet more than 2,500 years ago, Buddhist teachings named a truth that modern science now confirms through the practice of *mettā*, or loving-kindness. This practice was never meant only for others; it was designed to begin with the self. Because a mind at war with itself cannot heal. Self-compassion is not weakness; it is the foundation.

Research by Kristin Neff shows that people who practice self-compassion experience lower cortisol, reduced inflammation, and greater emotional resilience. Not because they lower their standards, but because they stop paying a biological penalty for self-attack.

Self-criticism activates the same fear centres in the brain as physical threats do. The body floods with stress. Clarity shuts down. Decision-making narrows. Self-compassion reverses this cascade: it activates the caregiving system, restores calm, and brings wise decision-making back online.

This is why *mettā* begins with the words, "May I be happy. May I be free from suffering." Not from selfishness, but from the recognition that a regulated nervous system is the prerequisite for real health, strength, and kindness.

Your inner voice is meant to heal, not hurt. When you stop fighting yourself and begin speaking with patience and understanding, fitness stops being a punishment and becomes a way of living. And that gentle shift, toward safety, awareness, and kindness, is where absolute freedom finally begins.

Reflection

These reflection pages are not a checklist. They are a pause. An invitation to set down the hammer of discipline, the measuring tape of worth, and the constant mental commentary, and finally listen. Not to rules. To yourself.

I. Remembering the "Golden Era"

There was a time when your body was not a project.

As a child, you moved because it felt electric; running until your lungs burned, stopping only when joy faded into a quiet hum of satisfaction. You ate because you were hungry. You stopped because you were full. Your body was not an object; it was home.

The Question: Can you remember when that neutrality disappeared? Was it a comment at a family table, a number spoken too loudly, a mirror that suddenly felt judgmental, or the trespasser of puberty that turned your body into a performance?

The Truth: You have spent years blaming willpower for biological changes that were never a failure of character. Your body did not betray you. It adapted.

II. Leaving the "Waiting Room"

Many of us live on layaway. We postpone joy; bright clothes, intimacy, confidence, beaches, ambition; until we become someone "better."

The Question: What are you waiting to do? And who taught you that joy must be earned through shrinking?

The Truth: The scale measures gravity, not goodness. It cannot quantify your courage, tenderness, creativity, or capacity for love.

III. Becoming the "Deaf Frog"

In the famous story, the frog who reaches the top succeeds not because he is stronger, but because he is deaf. He never absorbs the jeers telling him to stop.

The Question: Whose voices make health feel heavier: social media, relatives, your own inner narrator? Which opinions are you letting live rent-free in your body?

The Truth: Often, what needs changing is not your plate, but the voices you keep listening to.

IV. Choosing Curiosity Over the Hammer

Discipline has been taught as punishment. Slip once, and the day is "ruined."

The Question: What if you replaced judgment with curiosity? Instead of "I'm lazy," what if you said, "That's interesting; I skipped lunch, felt overwhelmed, and needed comfort"?

The Truth: Shame burns fast and leaves ash. Curiosity gathers information, and growth comes from understanding, not force.

V. Your Final Reflection

Put your phone face down. Close your eyes. Take a slow, fifteen-second breath.

If you were the last person on Earth, no mirrors, no opinions, no comparisons, how would you move your body today? Would you stretch, walk, rest, dance, or sit quietly? Would you eat to punish, impress, or nourish? Would your body be a temple for your soul, or a stage for someone else's approval?

Notice what arises without correcting it.

It is the moment you stop fighting yourself and begin listening.

Awareness & Breath Practices

These breathing rituals are not meant to be intense or complicated. They are simple ways to slow down, notice what is happening inside, and gently calm the nervous system. You do not need prior experience. A few minutes of attention is enough.

1. Nadi Shodhana (Alternate Nostril Breathing)

Duration: 3–5 minutes

When to use: When the mind feels restless, anxious, or emotionally unsettled

What it helps with: Mental balance, emotional steadiness

Sit comfortably with your spine upright. Close your eyes. Using one hand, gently close one nostril and breathe in through the other. Switch sides and breathe out. Continue alternating sides slowly. Keep the breath soft and unforced. This rhythm naturally settles scattered thoughts and brings a sense of inner balance.

2. Bhramari (Humming Bee Breath)

Duration: 2–3 minutes

When to use: During anxiety, irritation, or before sleep

What it helps with: Calming the nervous system, quieting the mind

Sit quietly and take a deep breath in through the nose. As you breathe out, make a soft humming sound with your mouth closed. Feel the vibration in your head and chest. Repeat gently. This vibration soothes the nervous system and helps release emotional tension that often leads to stress eating or restlessness.

3. Ujjayi (Victorious Breath)

Duration: 5 minutes

When to use: During stressful days or emotional pressure

What it helps with: Focus, emotional regulation

Breathe in and out through the nose while slightly tightening the throat to create a soft, ocean-like sound. Keep the breath slow and steady. Let the sound anchor your attention. This breath brings focus and helps reduce impulsive reactions during emotionally charged moments.

4. Sheetali / Sheetkari (Cooling Breath)

Duration: 2 minutes

When to use: During anger, agitation, or emotional overheating

What it helps with: Cooling emotions, calming urges

Breathe in gently through the mouth (either through a rolled tongue or slightly parted teeth), then breathe out slowly through the nose. Feel the cooling effect of the breath. This exercise is helpful when emotions feel heated or cravings feel urgent.

5. Kapalabhati (Gentle Movement)

Duration: 1–2 minutes

When to use: Morning or during mental heaviness

What it helps with: Mental clarity, renewed energy

Sit upright and breathe out gently but actively through the nose, allowing the inhale to happen naturally. Keep the movement light and relaxed. Used softly, this routine refreshes the mind without strain.

These approaches are not about doing more. They are about pausing. Even a few minutes of conscious breathing can shift how the body responds to stress and emotional eating. Over time, breath awareness becomes a steady support, helping you respond with calm rather than react on impulse.

Practical Awareness Toolkit

Here is a collection of concise tools, mental resets, and decision filters designed to help you cut through the mental noise of fitness, step out of pressure cycles, and reclaim a peaceful, rational relationship with your body.

You don't need to use everything. Pick one tool. Come back when needed.

1. Awareness Checks & Mental Reset

These practices interrupt spirals and bring you back to a state of neutrality.

The 15-Second Pause & Notice

When body anxiety hits, pause and ask: *"When did my body stop feeling neutral?"*

Was it a mirror, a comment, or scrolling? Name it; don't fix it. Awareness alone softens its power.

Fun activity: Turn this into a game called *Spot the Trigger*. Every time you catch one, you score a point.

The Sunlight Reset: Ask: *"Where did my eyes meet light today, the screen or the sky?"*

Step outside for 10 minutes. Natural light is a free mood and focus upgrade.

The Gratitude Scan: Before getting out of bed, name one thing your body did for you overnight: breathing, healing, or resting.

Appreciation builds discipline better than shame.

The Deaf Frog Technique: When faced with unhelpful comments, don't explain, defend, or engage. Keep hopping forward.

2. Decision Filters & Logical Audits

Use these to protect your mental bandwidth.

The Red-Flag Filter: Pause if you see:

- One-ingredient miracles
- Permanent results in 30 days
- Aesthetic hype without biology

The CEO vs. Toddler Check:

Before impulsive eating or reactive decisions, pause and ask: *"Am I tired, stressed, or underslept?"*

In this moment, think of your mind in two modes.

The **CEO** is your calm, rested, rational self; the part of you that can think clearly, plan ahead, and make balanced decisions.

The **toddler** is your exhausted, overwhelmed, reactive self;the state where emotions and impulses take over because the body needs care.

If the answer is yes, don't punish yourself or apply discipline. **Feed the body, rest it, and regulate it first.**

Toddlers shouldn't run the kitchen; and neither should decisions made from exhaustion.

Fun activity: Name your inner toddler. Giving it a name often makes it easier to notice impulsive moments without judgment.

The Taller Man Strategy

Ask: *"If no one were watching, how would I care for my body today?"*

Shift from approval to internal authority.

The Circle Check: Notice who makes healthy living feel lighter, and who makes it heavier. Adjust proximity gently.

3. Simple Daily Reminders

- **Confidence is a Track Record:** Small promises kept daily matter more than intensity.
- **The Gap Exists:** Results show up later than effort. Biology is working even when the evidence is quiet.
- **Count Non-Scale Victories:** Energy, focus, calmer moods; all wins.
- **Decision Fatigue Is Real:** Reduce choices with defaults and repeat meals.

Fun activity: Imagine a small jar. Each day you notice a non-scale win;energy, focus, calm; drop a coin into the jar.

When the jar feels "full enough" that week, give yourself a guilt-free rest day.

Awareness is not something you master.

It's something you **return to**, again and again.

Troubleshooting

Not every day will feel balanced; this table helps you respond with understanding when the body signals distress.

What You're Experiencing	What's Likely Happening	Awareness-Based Response (What to Do)
Restless or broken sleep	Your nervous system hasn't fully shifted out of "alert mode." Mental load, unresolved stress, or late-day stimulation may be keeping the body on guard.	Instead of forcing sleep, focus on *down-shifting*. Dim lights earlier. Reduce late-night decisions. Slow your breathing, especially the exhale. Ask: *What is my body still holding on to today?* Sleep improves when the body feels safe, not controlled.
Difficulty falling asleep despite fatigue	Physical tiredness is present, but mental or emotional processing is incomplete. The mind is still "working."	Create a gentle closing ritual for the day;quiet time, stillness, or silence. Avoid problem-solving at night. Let the body know the day is done before asking it to rest.

Sudden or intense cravings	Cravings are often signals of tiredness, stress, dehydration, or emotional overload;not hunger or lack of discipline.	Pause for a few seconds before acting. Ask: *Am I hungry, tired, stressed, or overstimulated?* Often, rest, hydration, or calming the mind reduces the craving naturally. Awareness interrupts the reflex.
Cravings despite eating enough	Stress hormones can override satiety signals, making the body seek quick comfort or stimulation.	Slow down. Ground yourself. Take a few deep breaths or step away from screens. Cravings lose power when the nervous system settles. You don't need to suppress them;just observe them.
Irritability or short temper	Accumulated fatigue, poor sleep, or constant self-pressure has made the nervous system reactive.	Reduce stimulation. Eat regularly. Step into natural light if possible. Notice internal self-criticism and soften it. Ask: *What am I carrying right now?* Mood stabilises with support, not force.
Low or flat mood	Emotional and physical energy may be depleted from prolonged	Lower the bar temporarily. Nourish consistency over intensity. Gentle movement, regular meals, and kindness toward yourself help restore

	stress or over-expectation.	balance faster than motivation ever will.

Lifestyle Cards

Life doesn't pause for routines.

These cards are for the days when schedules break, plans shift, and awareness feels harder to hold.

Use them as gentle reminders, not rules.

Travel Days

When routines dissolve somewhere between check-in and arrival.

- Treat travel as a holding pattern, not a performance.
- Eat before hunger becomes dramatic; hunger makes decisions louder.
- Choose food that feels recognisable, not impressive.
- Carry one tiny ritual through the journey:
- *sit to drink water, pause before the first bite, breathe once before eating.*
- Let one repeated action become your anchor when everything else is unfamiliar.
- Travel isn't chaos; it's compressed living. Cognition just needs less space.

Busy Workdays

When meals become accidental, the body runs on adrenaline.

- Stop waiting for a "proper break." Use transitions instead.

- Before opening a laptop. Before answering a call. Before leaving work.
- One slow breath is enough.
- Keep one meal that asks nothing of your brain.
- Familiar. Repeatable. Reliable.
- Eat like you're refuelling a teammate, not rewarding survival.
- Lower stimulation before eating; even a quiet minute changes digestion.
- Productivity improves when the body doesn't feel ignored.

Social Events & Eating Out

When food becomes emotion, memory, and negotiation.

- Decide *what you're saying yes to* before you arrive.
- One indulgence chosen consciously beats five eaten distractedly.
- Eat something simple beforehand; hunger distorts generosity.
- Sit angled toward people, not plates.
- Let conversation slow your eating instead of willpower.
- The event is the experience. Food is only one language of it.

Festivals, Illness, Poor Sleep

When structure collapses, and control feels tempting.

- Variety is overrated when the body is tired.
- Repetition creates safety.
- Warm. Simple. Regular.
- Let meals feel predictable when life isn't.
- Ask quietly before eating:
- *Is this about energy, comfort, or pause?*
- Not every need is hunger; some are nervous system requests.
- Consistency soothes more than discipline ever will.

When Conscious Noticing Slips

When you notice late, you judge faster.

- Late noticing is still noticing.
- Drop the commentary. Choose a neutral reset:
  - drink water, wash hands, or step outside
- Don't reply. Resume.
- Behaviour restores balance faster than thinking.
- Attunement doesn't vanish; it waits.

Epilogue

Close the book, but keep your hand on the page for just a moment. Feel the weight of it, then feel the weight of yourself. You are here, breathing & trying, caring, and still staying soft in a world that often demands you stay brittle. That quiet persistence says more about your character than any rigid routine ever could.

You were never failing. You were never lazy, broken, or lacking some mysterious spark of discipline. You were doing your best with a cultural narrative that taught you to push harder instead of listen closer. When life felt heavy or inconsistent, it wasn't because you didn't want it enough. It was because your system was crying out for understanding, not more pressure.

Most people finish a journey like this feeling a quiet panic about what they must "fix" by tomorrow morning. That tightness in your chest, the urgency to finally "get it right", is the very weight you are now invited to put down. This was never a project of correction; it was a process of homecoming. Beneath the static of rules and comparisons, your body has never been your saboteur. It has been your oldest friend, trying to communicate through the only language it has.

Nothing about you needed fixing. You needed to feel safe. Effort without kindness is just a slow-burning war, and no one can survive a fight forever. But when care replaces criticism, the internal landscape shifts. Movement becomes a way to inhabit your life, not a way to pay a debt. Rest becomes a form of wisdom, not a source of guilt.

What you are carrying forward is not a set of demands, but a new vocabulary of permission: Permission to pivot, be tender on the days that feel sharp, to trust your internal signals over the loud, external noise. This flexibility isn't a weakness; it is the marrow of true consistency, the kind that supports you rather than strains you.

You don’t need to be perfect to move forward; you only need to stay present. Some days will feel like a surge of power, others like a quiet retreat. Both belong. Listening is now your foundation. From this point on, change does not come from force; it grows from grace.

The finish line was a myth. Instead, there is just you, treating your body like an ally at last. That isn’t a small step. That is everything.

Verses Kindler Publication

Verses Kindler Publication

Reach us through our website -

https://www.verseskindlerpublication.com/

For more information visit our

Instagram or Facebook page.

9 789347 494468

Printed at Repro India Ltd.